Fighting Cancer with
Knowledge and Hope

Yale University Press Health & Wellness

A Yale University Press Health & Wellness book is an authoritative, accessible source of information on a health-related topic. It may provide guidance to help you lead a healthy life, examine your treatment options for a specific condition or disease, situate a health care issue in the context of your life as a whole, or address questions or concerns that linger after visits to your health care provider.

Fighting Cancer

with Knowledge & Hope

A Guide for Patients, Families, and Health Care Providers

RICHARD C. FRANK, MD

Illustrations by Gale V. Parsons

Yale University Press

New Haven & London

Published on the foundation established in memory of William Chauncey
Williams of the Class of 1822, Yale Medical School, and of William Cook
Williams of the Class of 1850, Yale Medical School.

Designed by Nancy Ovedovitz and set in Simoncini Garamond type by
Tseng Information Systems, Inc. Printed in the United States of America.

Library of Congress Cataloging-in-Publication Data
Frank, Richard C., MD.
Fighting cancer with knowledge and hope : a guide for patients, families, and health care
providers / Richard C. Frank ; illustrations by Gail V. Parsons.
p.   cm. —(Yale University Press health & wellness)
Includes bibliographical references and index.
ISBN 978-0-300-15102-2 (paperbound : alk. paper) —
ISBN 978-0-300-14926-5 (clothbound : alk. paper)
1. Cancer—Popular works. I. Title. II. Series.
[DNLM: 1. Neoplasms—Popular Works. QZ 201 F828f 2009]
RC263.F695 2009
616.99′4—dc22   2008048917

A catalogue record for this book is available from the British Library.

This paper meets the requirements of ANSI/NISO z39.48-1992 (Permanence of Paper).

10   9   8   7   6   5   4   3   2   1

To my patients, who have granted
me the great privilege of being their
oncologist

In memory of my mother, Nina Frank,
for a lifetime of encouragement,
inspiration, and supreme love

The journey of a thousand miles begins with a single step.
—Lao Tzu

Contents

Foreword

Fighting Cancer with Knowledge and Hope provides you with the information you need to survive cancer. But above everything else, Dr. Frank gives you the wisdom to knock out the despair and depression brought on by cancer. He gives you a needed dose of tranquillity.

Dr. Frank does something very important in this book, and that is to truly demystify cancer. I am not in favor of using that word without an explanation. Demystification evaporates the mystery of cancer, so that you can see clearly and stand courageously wherever you are. Fear disappears, because you finally come to understand the old syllogism: "A human being is mortal. I am a human being. Therefore, I am mortal."

Being mortal can be a blessing if we believe an old Greek myth. In that story, a man who did not want to die begged the gods to grant him immortality and eternal youth. Tired of his pestering, they gave him his request. He grew old, watched his family die, and saw his friends pass away. The people he loved were gone, leaving him lonely and in despair. He again begged the gods, this time to allow him to die. They agreed, and he died the happiest man on earth.

In James Hilton's novel *Lost Horizon* (as well as in the film starring

Ronald Coleman) the strangers who landed in the Himalayan valley of Shangri-La became bored with eternal youth. They escaped and thus completed their destiny as human beings to become old and die.

Cancer is the hands of the gods, reminding us that we are mortal. Dr. Frank's book is the kind hand of a brilliant oncologist who lets you know that it is not yet your time to die, that you can still enjoy your old age, that you can still live without pain, that when you have to go, you can go painlessly, leaving your loved ones in peace, having completed many unfinished projects and business.

Ironically, cancer cells don't want to die; they want to be immortal. They want to obliterate human destiny and to reproduce endlessly by the billions. When the bells strike the final hour for their human host, they all die as the body enters into the kingdom of not-this-world, into the kingdom of eternal peace, the kingdom of a dream without nightmares.

The great Peruvian poet César Vallejo wrote, "After all, one is half-dead, and half-alive, in this life." This is probably true; however, cancer can save you from this human condition and show you a good side effect. It makes you shout, "After all, I am still alive!" And then, knowing you may die, you start living intensely. If you are a good person, you become a better person. If you are not good, you become good. Your life instinct becomes sharp as a knife. Dr. Frank shows the enormous energy spent by the human body in fighting cancer for twenty, thirty, or more years. This concentrated life force, like a huge army, works to defeat cancer for a few or many years of life, with the help of surgery, radiation therapy, and the wonder drugs of chemotherapy and targeted treatments. Their side effects are nothing compared with what you get from them: a transitory reprieve from the way of all flesh.

If you are not a cancer patient, and you carry in your genes the defect that will strike you down sooner or later, this book will give you the strength you need for the big fight.

I have read many books about cancer, from Dr. Linus Pauling's *Cancer and Vitamin C,* Dr. Virginia Livingston-Wheeler's *The Conquest of Cancer,* and Dr. Max Gerson's *A Cancer Therapy* to Claudia I. Henschke's

Lung Cancer, Dr. Carolyn D. Runowicz and Dr. Sheldon H. Cherry's *The Answer to Cancer,* Adam Wishart's *One in Three.* This book, however, stands out from the crowd. Dr. Frank shows what is happening in that mysterious world of cancer research, of anticancer drugs that are being discovered and tested every day, and of that incomprehensible and baffling world of genetics and cancer.

I know you will feel as I do, that this book produces knowledge, hope, and optimism.

Edmundo Bendezu, PhD
Professor of Spanish Literature
University of Nebraska
Lincoln, Nebraska
San Marcos University
Lima, Peru

Preface

Cancer is a frightening and complicated illness. Those affected by it face a series of new challenges after hearing the words "It's cancer." On being diagnosed, most people feel alone, as if nobody can truly relate to their innermost fears. They will receive advice from well-meaning friends and family and will seek answers in magazines and books and on the Internet. They will meet with specialists and strive to get the best medical care possible. They will challenge themselves to eat right, exercise right, live right, think positively, accept treatments diligently, and suffer side effects bravely. And they will often strive to contain their fears from their loved ones and caregivers.

Although the chances of beating cancer improve every year, the road to survival is often not easy. A cancer patient may need to undergo surgery and suffer pain and an altered body image and receive radiation treatments that may cause mouth sores, diarrhea, or skin irritation. They may be treated with chemotherapy and fight to keep their bodies intact while confronting hair loss, weakness, lowered immunity, and strange reactions to potent drugs.

Cancer patients may travel long distances or make frequent trips for their treatments, battling inconvenience and a diminished quality of life. They may face new financial burdens to pay for their medical care. They may choose to participate in research studies and experience rollercoaster fear and hope as a result of receiving unproven but promising treatments.

All cancer patients will, throughout their cancer journeys, suffer the anxiety of not knowing if their treatments are working or for how long their treatments will work or if they will survive their cancer.

With all these cancer-related issues to think about, it may come as a revelation to many battling cancer that throughout their cancer odyssey, they will rarely think clearly about the disease itself. Cancer patients think a great deal about what cancer is doing to their lives and to their bodies, and understandably so. They also concentrate on their choice of treatment and caregivers.

But why do so few focus healing thoughts on the very disease that has become the focus of their lives? Based on the multitude of questions I field daily from cancer patients and their loved ones, there is clearly a burning desire to better understand the cancer process. I believe the main reason that many people feel overwhelmed when it comes to trying to make sense of cancer is that few people know what the disease is or how to think about it.

The very thing that has turned a person's life upside down is a mystery to them.

My motivation to write this book stems directly from the words of my patients—more specifically, the burning questions that so many of them have and rarely get answered to their satisfaction. When first diagnosed, most patients want to know why they got cancer and if it could have been caught earlier. After deciding on the most appropriate treatment, many want to know how those treatments work and, if they should fail to control the cancer, why they failed. The answers, of course, are specific to each individual, and in most cases, accurate answers are truly not available. Yet after hearing the frustrated words of a vibrant woman dying from stomach cancer—"What the hell is this beast inside of me? I feel like I have no control over anything that is going on inside my body"—I knew that more information needed to be made available to those who want answers or at least as much knowledge as possible.

The main goals of this book are to enable you to appreciate:

1. What cancer is and how it grows;
2. How oncologists determine the best treatment for each patient and what the different treatment strategies are; and
3. How to visualize cancer treatments at work in the body.

My purpose is to impart knowledge and a fresh perspective on some of the most complicated but essential aspects of cancer that have thus far received little attention. These include descriptions of the development, growth, and death of cancer (with treatment), written in a way that any reader without previous scientific knowledge will understand. I also include those aspects of practical cancer management that I have found most important in my day-to-day practice, such as how to cope in the face of a poor prognosis, facing fears of chemotherapy, and the distinction between chemotherapy and newer, targeted medicines. I hope you will find, as one of my patients did, that "reading this book is like having a conversation with your oncologist."

By reading this book, you will come to understand that *no two cancers are exactly alike.* Two individuals with the exact same cancer diagnosis will almost certainly experience their diseases differently. Their cancers will grow at different rates, affect their bodies in distinct ways, and respond uniquely to the same treatments (one person's cancer may disappear with a treatment, whereas another's may grow while receiving the same treatment). Yet despite these differences and complexities, all cancers share features that explain why a cell anywhere in the body can became a cancer cell. Further, these shared biological roots explain why many of the same treatments are being applied to treat a wide range of cancers, such as angiogenesis inhibitor therapies that alter blood flow to a tumor. Thus, regardless of the type of cancer you may have or are interested in, the principles described in this book are directly relevant to it.

In Part 1, I draw on actual patient case histories, from my hematology and oncology practice, to explain the behavior of cancer in the body, how the different cancers are staged, and how oncologists estimate curability. Current thinking about the causes of cancer and the best means to prevent it is also covered.

In Part 2, I cover why oncologists recommend a particular sequence of surgery, chemotherapy, and/or radiation. Next, I explore how the major forms of cancer-fighting drugs (chemotherapy, targeted therapies, and hormone therapies) work to shut down cancer growth. Illustrations accompany the discussions to cement deeper levels of comprehension; they help you visualize and capture with your "mind's eye" the essence of how treatments attack cancer. No longer will you feel like an innocent bystander, blindly accepting bewildering medicines for an impenetrable disease.

In the final chapter, you will learn the coping strategies recommended by those who have survived cancer so that you are in the right frame of mind to face the disease.

This book will be useful as an aid during various aspects of your treatment. While receiving chemotherapy or radiation therapy, you can use the pictures showing how that treatment works so that you can guide the therapy with your mind. The visualization of cancer dying and the body healing is an important tool because it enables you to engage your mental energies on the task at hand; doing so will promote a sense of calm in dealing with the disease.

If you are a cancer patient, I must tell you that I do not know if focusing your thoughts on cancer will help you live longer. But with a greater understanding of the disease you are battling, you will feel more in control of your situation. And with more control, you will be more relaxed and better able to cope with the many ups and downs that every cancer patient experiences.

I wish you long life and victory over cancer.

Richard C. Frank, MD

Acknowledgments

I am especially indebted to the following individuals: Nancy and Robert Biewen, for believing in this work early in its development, for their continuous input and advice, and for their tremendous spirit and love; Anthony Coscia, MD, for his superior editing skills and clinical wisdom; my agent, Jacques de Spoelberch, for embracing this book and giving me the confidence to complete it; Jean Thomson Black, executive editor at Yale University Press, for her vision, integrity, and steadfast support of this work; Gale V. Parsons, for applying her unique artistic talent and for being an absolute pleasure to work with; and the late Charles Sovek, artist, friend, and mentor to Gale and me.

I am so grateful to the many talented and giving individuals who provided essential feedback to me as I wrote this book: Elizabeth April-Fritz, Carol Avery, EdD, RNC, Edmundo Bendezu, PhD, Mary Ann Bendezu, Melinda Brockwell, RN, Rose Buzzutto, RN, Peter Clarke, Raymond Comenzo, MD, Michele Dailey, LMFT, Bridget DeBartolomeo, RN, Nancy Gennaro, MSW, William Hale, MD, Nancy and Richard Husta, Andrew Jaffe, Francoise Jaffe, PhD, MSW, Ann Jakubowski, MD, Helen Kandel-Hyman, Mary-Ellen Loncto, RN, Jennifer Long, APRN, Ellen

Matloff, MS, William Mitchell, Michele Montano, Kesav Nair, MD, Rita Ort, RN, Pradip Pathare, MD, Martha and Mark Potter, Florence Price, Phyllis Osterman, Margaret Raleigh, Jerry Roberts, Christopher Roule, Samir Safwat, Seema Sanghavi, MD, William Sikov, MD, Valerie Solis, RN, Phyllis and Stephen Steinbrecher, Lynn and Bill Thompson, Linda Versea, APRN, and Richard Zelkowitz, MD. It is certainly not enough, but thank you all very much!

Special thanks to the staff at Yale University Press, especially Laura Jones Dooley, senior manuscript editor, for her excellent editing of this book, as well as Jenya Weinreb, managing editor, and Matthew Laird. I also wish to thank Jill Golrick, head of library sciences at Norwalk Hospital, for always being so helpful.

I gratefully acknowledge the tremendous work of the staff of the Whittingham Cancer Center, the oncology section of the Norwalk Medical Group, the 6E inpatient and outpatient oncology units of Norwalk Hospital, and the Mid-Fairfield Hospice. Your attention and devotion to the individual is what great cancer care is all about. It is my privilege to be a part of such a caring environment.

A note of thanks also goes to Ms. Diane Blum, MSW, Executive Director of CancerCare. CancerCare (www.cancercare.org) is a national nonprofit organization that provides free, professional support services to anyone affected by cancer, a very worthy endeavor for which a portion of the royalties earned on this book will be donated.

Most important, a most loving thank-you to my wife, Miriam, for her love and support, many insightful comments, and putting up with me at all times, especially as I wrote this book in the thicket of raising two small children. And to those beautiful children, Adam and Sam, thank you for your wonder and smiles and for giving us such pride and joy. Finally, to my sister, Shawn, social worker par excellence, sister without rival, thank you for your great inner strength, for a lifetime of friendship and caring, and for your insight into the needs of cancer survivors.

Fighting Cancer with Knowledge and Hope

Part I

Exposing Cancer

I
Understanding Cancer

When I first laid eyes on Alice, I could tell she was in trouble. "Trouble" for me, a medical oncologist, means that a patient is sick from cancer and in urgent need of treatment. But like so many patients whom I meet for the first time, Alice was not even sure she had cancer. So "trouble" also means that I faced a daunting task: I had to explain to Alice (and her family) what cancer is, why it may have arisen, what it was doing to her body, which treatments were recommended, how those treatments worked, and how she could cope when her world was crashing in on her—all this in about an hour.

Furthermore, I needed to convey this information with great empathy and sensitivity, never forgetting that although my brain may sleep, eat, and breathe cancer, the cancer "lingo" is completely foreign to a person newly diagnosed with the disease.

As I present my assessment of a cancer situation to a new patient and family, my senses enter a state of heightened awareness: I continually monitor the body language of my listeners to discern if I am making myself understood, if my words are too strong or not strong enough, or if I should stop the flow of words to allow the necessary flow of emotions. I have taken to using a marker board, like a mini-lecture, to write out the technical words and details. As with so many other oncologists, there is no need to ask me, "What would you do if I were your brother, wife, or mother?" Please understand that this is always a given.

As Alice walked into my office for a consultation, her husband and daughter were close behind. She was clearly exhausted, gasped slightly with each breath, and, after spotting the chair nearest to me, slumped into it. She exuded a soft, sincere demeanor, though she was obviously weighed down by worry.

Alice gathered herself as I introduced myself, and then she asked me in a sweet, perplexed voice, "Doctor, what's wrong with me? I am so tired I can't even climb a flight of stairs. My stomach is bloated and I hardly eat anymore. Am I dying?"

Before I met with Alice, I had reviewed her medical records. She had recently seen her internist, complaining of several months of unremitting fatigue, loss of appetite, and shortness of breath with exertion. Her doctor had ordered CT scans of her chest, abdomen, and pelvis. These showed a large tumor on one of her ovaries, many other tumors throughout her abdomen, and smaller tumors throughout her lungs. He ordered a biopsy of one of the abdominal tumors, and it revealed a diagnosis of ovarian cancer. The tumors throughout Alice's abdomen and chest indicated that she had the most advanced stage of that cancer. A blood marker of ovarian cancer, named CA-125, was many times above the normal range, consistent with this diagnosis.

When Alice walked through the office doorway, I knew immediately that all her symptoms were caused by cancer. The sheer burden of having tumors involving so much of her body was exhausting her. The disease was competing with the rest of her body for vital nutrients, and the cancer was siphoning most of these away. The tumors in her lungs were interfering with the ability of her lungs to transfer oxygen to her bloodstream for delivery throughout her body; this accounted for her shortness of breath. The many tumors in her abdomen were causing her belly to swell and taking away her appetite.

I began to talk to her. "I can see that you are suffering. Your breathing appears labored to me, and I can tell that you must be struggling just to get through the day." With this, she nodded and began to weep. But this was a cry of relief; someone had finally explained why her condition was deteriorating so fast. "I will explain exactly what is wrong with you and tell you what we need to do to get you feeling better," I said. "But I want to start off by saying that you will very likely be feeling better soon." With that, she relaxed and started to breathe more easily.

I explained what her CT scans showed and what the pathology report indicated. I told her she had ovarian cancer and that it had spread from her ovary to her abdomen and into her lungs, which classified it as stage IV. I explained how the extent of the cancer was causing all her symptoms and that if we could shrink it, she would begin to feel better.

"Do I need chemo?" she asked. "I'm afraid of that, I don't know if my body can stand it." "Yes," I replied, "we do need to use chemotherapy. But since most of your symptoms are due to the growth of the cancer, once we stop that growth with chemotherapy, you will actually feel better. There certainly will be side effects from treatment, but we will monitor you closely for them and try to prevent as many as possible." Alice did not voice further opposition to the chemotherapy. She understood that she would be fighting for her life.

"The standard recommended treatment," I continued, "is two chemotherapy drugs, called Taxol and carboplatin, which are administered intravenously every three weeks. We are also participating in a study to determine whether adding a new medication to this standard treatment improves the outcome." We discussed the short-term and long-term side effects of chemotherapy and went over the pros and cons of participating in the clinical trial. I told her that after our meeting, she would visit one of our oncology nurses, who would further explain what to expect and how to prepare for treatment.

"Why can't it just all be cut out?" Alice asked. "For most cases of ovarian cancer," I replied, "surgery actually is the first step of treatment. But in your situation, because the cancer has spread outside of the abdomen and is causing so many symptoms, we need to attack it with a treatment that will shrink the cancer wherever it is growing in your body; the disease is too extensive at this point for surgery to be effective. So we need to start with chemotherapy and reserve surgery for a later date."

I inquired about her family history and whether other family members had been affected by cancer, in particular breast and ovarian cancer. When she answered yes, we discussed the need for genetic testing, which she wanted to do at another time. We talked briefly about her family life, habits, and spirituality as I tried to get a sense of the person.

After I answered the questions Alice and her family had, I told them about the counseling services for patients and families at our center: group counseling, in which those who have traveled or are traveling a similar road can share experiences; and individual counseling, in which patients can privately express to an experienced therapist their feelings, fears, and needs as a cancer patient and survivor.

We ended our first meeting exhausted. But we also ended it as partners, hopeful that Alice's condition would improve. I knew that we had covered a tremendous amount of new and complicated information and that Alice would probably remember only a part of it. I reassured her that we would have ample time, in future meetings together, to go over what we had discussed.

My meeting with Alice and her family highlights the essential information that any patient must find out when he or she is diagnosed with cancer. The following list summarizes this information.

When First Diagnosed: What You Need to Learn

- ◆ the type of cancer
- ◆ the stage (extent) of the cancer
- ◆ whether cure is to be expected
- ◆ possible environmental or genetic influences that may have predisposed you to develop cancer
- ◆ important aspects of the cancer, called "prognostic factors" (see chapter 2), that may help determine your prognosis

- whether you have other medical problems that may affect your choice of treatment
- recommended treatments, their schedules, and their duration
- side effects from treatment (likely and less likely), both short term and long term
- what can be done to prevent or minimize those side effects, should they occur
- other treatment options, such as (1) a different but equally effective chemotherapy drug whose side effects may better meet your needs (for example, less hair loss or a reduced chance of numbness in the hands and feet, called peripheral neuropathy), and (2) a different sequence of chemotherapy, radiation, or surgery than is being proposed and the merits of the different approaches
- if a clinical trial (research study) testing new ways to treat the cancer is available and the pros and cons of participating in the study
- what the strategy might be if the first therapy does not control the cancer
- whether a second opinion is advisable (initially or at a future time)
- how the treatment costs will be covered
- a review of the medications, vitamins, and supplements you may already be taking
- where to find counseling and support groups to help you and your loved ones cope with the many emotional and life challenges posed by cancer

These essential topics are covered in later chapters. First I wish to focus on the disease itself and answer the deceptively simple question, "What is cancer?"

Alice's story provides one answer: *All of the above is cancer.* Cancer is all the physical and emotional upheaval that a person's body and mind must endure in response to an "invasion from within" of bizarre collections of cells that form troubling growths called tumors. From a medical point of view, cancer can be defined another way:

> What is Cancer? *Cancer is a disease caused by the growth and spread in our bodies of cells that do not know how to die.*

The Three Essential Properties of Cancer

All cancers begin with the conversion of one cell from a normal state into a cancerous state. During this process, which in most cases takes many years, the changing cell acquires three main properties that distinguish it as a cancer cell. These three essential properties are the defining characteristics of the disease. Normal cells have none of these properties. The three properties are:

1. An unlimited capacity for growth
2. An inability to die
3. An ability to spread (from the site of origin)

To know these properties is to appreciate the very nature of cancer. They define how well a cancer grows and survives in the body, and they largely determine how curable any particular cancer is. It is extremely important to realize, however, that the power and extent of each property is different for each cancer. Some cancers grow slowly, others quickly; some have a great capacity to spread throughout the body, others a more limited ability to do so. *Just as every person is unique, so is every cancer.* This is why I caution patients that the information they receive about other people with cancer will probably not relate to their case.

AN UNLIMITED CAPACITY FOR GROWTH

The growth of cancer is very much on the minds of all those affected by this disease: patients, physicians, and researchers.

When a cancer patient wonders how long it has been from the time his or her cancer first started to when it was diagnosed, he or she is asking about the growth rate of the cancer. Another way to phrase this question is: "How fast is the cancer growing?" When a patient asks if the cancer is in "remission," he or she is really asking if the cancer has stopped growing and, more to the point, started to shrink. On the other hand, if the patient is told that the cancer has "relapsed," then it means the cancer is growing again.

> The Meaning of Remission. *There are two main types of remission: partial or complete. In a partial remission, the cancer shrinks in size by at least 30 percent; in a complete remission, the cancer becomes undetectable. In the past, cancer doctors and researchers believed that only treatments that achieved remission could benefit patients. However, some newer cancer treatments, called targeted therapies (discussed in chapters 6 and 7), not only improve quality of life but prolong life merely by "freezing" or stabilizing the growth of cancer (without necessarily shrinking tumors); this has led to a new mindset about the goals of therapy. Especially for cancers that are not considered curable, prolonged stabilization of the cancer can be as worthy a goal as obtaining remission.*

Oncologists (physicians with advanced training and certification in the medical care of people with cancer) have the same concerns as patients, but with a focus on how the health of their patients is or will be affected by cancer growth. For each patient, oncologists weigh several factors to assess and anticipate the growth potential of a cancer. These include: (1) examining the pathology report, which can indicate the aggressiveness of the cancer and its potential to return after treatment; (2) determining how rapidly any symptoms caused by the disease have developed; and (3) assessing the extent of the cancer as determined by imaging tests (CT scans, MRIs, bone scans, and PET scans) and blood tests.

Some types of cancer generate a protein, called a "tumor marker," that is released into the bloodstream and can be measured through a simple blood test. Although very elevated tumor marker levels often indicate an aggressive cancer, these tests are conducted primarily to track the progress of treatment (as a cancer is successfully treated, its tumor marker will fall). The main tumor markers are:

Major cancer tumor markers (blood tests)

Tumor marker	Cancer
AFP, HCG	testicular, liver (AFP only)
CEA	colorectal
CA 15-3, CA 27-29	breast
CA 19-9	pancreatic, biliary tract
CA-125	ovarian
PSA	prostate
M-protein; free light chains	multiple myeloma
LDH	lymphoma
Beta-2 microglobulin	myeloma, lymphoma

Oncologists process all this information to determine if a cancer is fast or slow growing and if it has a high or low potential to spread to other organs. *Oncologists must see the full cancer landscape for each patient, that which the affected person could not possibly see.* Following these assessments, the oncologist makes recommendations as to whether treatment should be started urgently (the same day) or in the near term (in a few days or weeks), or whether treatment can be deferred based on the future behavior of the cancer (that is, no treatment is necessary at present). For example, a person who experiences sudden back pain and is found to have a rapidly growing tumor that is pressing on the spinal cord requires urgent treatment to alleviate pain and prevent paralysis. In contrast, a seventy-five-year-old man with a slow-growing prostate cancer that is not causing any symptoms may never need the cancer treated. All of these clinical lines of thought revolve around the growth properties of the cancer in question. For each patient, the growth assessment of the cancer is best understood through discussions with the oncologist.

Cancer researchers are also focused on growth as they work to dis-

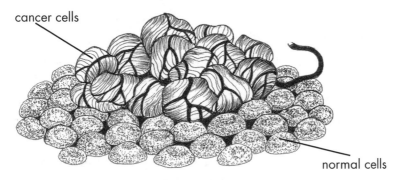

cancer cells

normal cells

Fig. 1. *The growth of cancer*
Normal cells form an organized pattern in the body, whereas cancer cells
grow on top of one another as they multiply. Illustration © Gale V. Parsons.

cover new and better ways of treating cancer. Scientists study the molecules inside cancer cells that stimulate them to multiply and grow. By
understanding how these important molecules work, researchers can
develop drugs that will block them from functioning. The hope is that
interfering with these critical targets will cause the cancer cells to die.
These growth targets and the drugs designed to block them are discussed later.

We've established that growth is central to thinking about cancer. But
what does it mean for cancer to grow, and to grow in an unlimited way?
What actually is growing? The answer is the number of cancer cells. All
cancers start with one cell, and that cell multiplies to form the tumors
that are ultimately detected. One cell becomes two cells. These two cells
then duplicate themselves to become four cells, which multiply to eight
cells, and so on, until there is an entire population of cells (fig. 1).

It is generally thought that one billion cancer cells need to have
formed before a cancer can be detected. This is the number of cells
present in a one-centimeter tumor (nearly a third of an inch). The ability
to detect cancer when far fewer cells are present is a high priority of
cancer research.

While the growth of cancer cells is certainly a bad thing, the growth
of healthy cells is of course, necessary for our bodies to function properly. The difference between normal cell growth and cancer cell growth

is that normal growth is always precisely timed and controlled. For example, when a human fetus is developing, cell growth is explosive because one fertilized egg must give rise to the trillions of cells that ultimately compose a body. Yet the process of making the heart, brain, or any other organ is tightly regulated: cells stop growing once the correct organ pattern is laid down. In fact, when an organ reaches maturity, most of its cells lose the capacity to multiply. This is why our heart cannot replace damaged cardiac muscle after a heart attack and why our bodies cannot heal a spinal cord injury by making new nerve tissue.

Mature adult organs have a limited capacity to regenerate, with the exception of the liver, the inner lining of the intestines, and the bone marrow. Fetal tissue, on the other hand, has the full capacity to form new cells, which is why fetal stem cells (the cells with the greatest regenerative capacity) are being studied as a way to help victims of numerous illnesses and injuries, such as Parkinson's disease and spinal cord damage. The hope is that if fetal stem cells are implanted in an environment of nerves, for example, they will sprout new nerve cells to replace the damaged ones.

The major exception to the rule that adult cells do not multiply freely is cancer. Cancer cells derive from the cells of our fully formed organs, but they have found a way, through genetic mutation (explained in chapter 4), to bypass the natural brakes on cell growth. By sustaining alterations to DNA elements that control growth, cancer cells acquire a limitless ability to multiply. In addition, they become impervious to the checks and balances that our bodies have developed to restrain rebellious cells.

Fortunately, other factors limit the size of any tumor (cancers do not just grow and grow). Yet because of this powerful growth engine, cancer must be fought with strong treatments, such as chemotherapy and radiation, that attempt to stop this growth in its tracks. The differences in growth between normal cells and cancer cells can be exploited by chemotherapy and radiation, which preferentially attack the actively dividing cancer cells.

Can we determine the exact growth rate of a cancerous tumor? No.

At this time, there is no precise way for doctors to assess the growth rate of a particular cancer. The technology has not yet been developed. Moreover, such a measure would be a complicated affair, because cancers change their growth patterns as they increase in size (the rate of growth slows as they get bigger) and as they are exposed to treatments (which attempt to slow the rate of growth considerably). But if such a test were available, it would undoubtedly show that no two cancers grow at exactly the same rate. Across the vast spectrum of cancer and its many different types is an even greater range of growth rates. Some cancers grow fast, and some grow slowly. This rate relates mainly to the specific constellation of molecules that define each cancer (no two cancers are exactly alike). For most tumors, changes in size are a balance between factors that promote growth and others that limit growth, such as the available supply of blood and nutrients. In fact, some cancers grow so slowly that they remain the same size from month to month or even from year to year.

> *Although cancer is commonly thought of as a disease caused by cells "growing out of control" or "running amok," this simple conception of cancer is inaccurate.*

I have been caring for Don, a seventy-five-year-old man who recently received his first treatments for a non-Hodgkin's lymphoma (a cancer of an immune cell called a lymphocyte) that was diagnosed when he was fifty years old. Throughout much of the intervening twenty-five years, Don experienced what we call "stable disease." He carried on with his life with his cancer untreated. Periodic CT scans showed that the tumors were either the same size or only slightly larger from one year to the next.

Stable disease is when a person and his or her cancer live in peaceful coexistence—a period when the cancer is not growing much and the body's natural defenses can keep it in check. It also implies that the cancer is not causing the patient any symptoms, so he or she is not ill.

In the past year, however, Don's lymphoma grew more rapidly, a situation termed "progressive disease," which necessitated his treatment. Yet despite the diagnosis of cancer many years ago, Don has lived a full and active life before, during, and after its treatment.

The message of Don's story is that many cancers do not grow like wildfire. For sure, some do develop rapidly, such as the blood cell cancers acute leukemia and high-grade lymphoma and aggressive forms of the more common organ-derived cancers (see chapter 3). But for others, the dominant problem with cancer cells is not that they are growing out of control and forming large tumors but that they just won't die once they are formed. This leads us to the second essential property of cancer.

AN INABILITY TO DIE

It is written in Ecclesiastes, "To every thing there is a season . . . A time to be born, and a time to die." So it is with the cells of our body; so it is not for cancer cells.

Each cell is born with a finite, predetermined life span. Some cells are meant to live for just a few hours, others (such as our brain cells) to survive all our lives. In addition, as cells undergo subtle changes as part of the normal aging process and experience the wear and tear of life in the body, some accumulate sufficient damage that requires their removal and replacement. In order to maintain just the right balance of cells at all times, our bodies have developed an elaborate biological system. This system clears out defective cells, eliminates diseased ones, and removes older ones to make room for new ones. The system actually operates inside each cell that is to be eliminated. When a cell's "time is up," a large network of molecules within the cell, which had been maintained in an inactive, or "locked-down" state, is liberated. This sets in motion a cascade of chemical reactions that cause the cell's various internal parts to dissolve, leading to cell suicide; the cell breaks into smaller units that are carted off by scavenger immune cells. To ensure that the process of cell suicide never fails, Mother Nature has programmed it

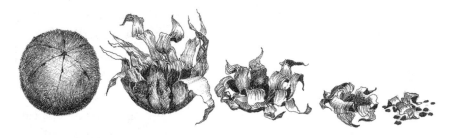

Fig. 2. *The death of cancer*
A cancer cell in the process of dying, called "programmed cell death" or apoptosis. Illustration © Gale V. Parsons.

into our genes—that is, the DNA of nearly every living cell has within it the potential to take a dagger to the heart of that very cell. The process is called "programmed cell death," or apoptosis. In Greek, *apoptosis* means "falling off" or "dropping off," as in leaves from a tree or petals from a flower (fig. 2).

Apoptosis is rarely mentioned in mainstream media reports on science and medicine. This is unfortunate, because apoptosis plays a pivotal role during the development of animals and in their health and disease. For example, when a tadpole metamorphoses into a frog, its tail disappears because the tail cells undergo apoptosis. To sculpt the fingers and toes of the developing human fetus out of an amorphous mound of tissue, the cells between the individual digits undergo apoptosis and fade away. When a virus infects us, it survives in our bodies by living inside certain cells; to rid the body of the virus, our immune system forces the infected cells to undergo apoptosis, taking the virus down with them. Slowly debilitating diseases of the nervous system, such as Parkinson's disease and Alzheimer's disease, are characterized by the progressive loss of nerve cells in the brain, which undergo premature apoptosis.

Why is apoptosis so important to cancer? The answer is that cancer cells have a diminished ability to undergo apoptosis. That is, they resist the signals that tell a normal cell to die. They ignore their programmed life span and fail to commit suicide when they are old; they live on in the face of injury after wear and tear; they resist the immune system's attempt to delete them. Cancer cells can do all these things because they have an altered genetic program of apoptosis wrought by changes (mutations) in their DNA. The result is that, inside a cancer cell, the programmed cell death apparatus is in perpetual lockdown.

If left to their own devices, most cancer cells in any tumor would fail to die and the tumor mass would keep growing. Fortunately, cancer cells' resistance to apoptosis is relative; many cancers will undergo apoptosis when targeted by anticancer treatments. As we know, some cancers are more successfully treated than others. Curable cancers (for example, testicular cancer and Hodgkin lymphoma) rapidly undergo apoptosis upon treatment, whereas those that are difficult to cure fail to undergo total apoptosis in response to treatment (treatment resistance is explained in chapter 7). Causing the death of cancers through apoptosis is a major goal of cancer therapies and of course the main desire of cancer patients.

In sum, the capacity to die exists within all cells. In nature, life and death are equally important and must be in balance. Normal cells obey the internal commands of their predetermined life span or the external cues of the body and commit suicide when so directed. Cancer cells disregard these signals and resist apoptosis. They have acquired an inability to die; the goal of cancer treatments is to overcome this barrier to their destruction.

AN ABILITY TO SPREAD (FROM THE SITE OF ORIGIN)

"Was the cancer caught in time?" This is one of the first and most important questions patients ask when they are diagnosed with cancer. With this question, they are asking if their cancer was detected before it had a chance to spread to other parts of the body (a process called "metastasis"). It is commonly thought that if a cancer has not metastasized, then it is curable, but if it has metastasized, then it is not curable. For many cancers, this is true, but there are many exceptions, so it is important to avoid generalizations. For example, if lung cancer has spread to the liver or brain, then it is rarely curable (note that I did not say "never curable" because there are people who have beaten advanced lung cancer). In contrast, testicular cancer that has spread to the same locations is potentially curable, as evidenced by the superhuman cyclist Lance Armstrong, who overcame testicular cancer that spread to his brain.

Another common reason to ask if the cancer was caught early enough is that many people have fears about chemotherapy and hope that if their cancer is contained, then locally directed therapies, such as surgery or radiation, will be all that is required for them to beat their cancer. This fear is understandable because chemotherapy drugs are strong medicines that can cause serious side effects. But extreme aversions to chemotherapy need to be dispelled because these medicines save lives. And chemotherapy administration today causes far fewer side effects than in the past. Many cancer patients today can live reasonably normal lives, even work and enjoy leisure activities, while undergoing chemotherapy treatments. I am always amazed at how many patients in our outpatient infusion room are eating away while chemotherapy drips into their arm through an intravenous line. Many have a bagel in one hand, an IV pole in the other, and are scooting around talking to others to pass the time. This could not have happened twenty years ago, when nausea and vomiting wracked patients and kept them in their hospital beds.

To describe how cancer spreads, I need to introduce some medical terms. The organ where a cancer originates is called the "primary" site. The breast is the primary site in breast cancer, the prostate the primary site for prostate tumors, and so on. For example, a breast cancer begins in a breast cell that becomes transformed into a cancer cell and multiplies into a tumor that becomes detectable. This same process is repeated during the birth of every cancer. The main primary sites of origin for cancers affecting men and women are discussed in chapter 3.

The locations in the body where a cancer spreads are called "metastatic" or secondary sites. Metastatic sites develop when individual cancer cells leave the primary tumor mass and travel to another location in the body, where they grow into tumors. Although a cancer can spread to virtually any part of the body, each type is associated with certain "preferred" distant sites. Knowledge of these sites guides the initial assessment of the extent of disease (called the "staging workup"; see chapter 2). For example, a patient with newly diagnosed lung cancer will undergo: a CT scan of the chest to search for spread of the disease to other parts of the lungs as well as lymph nodes in the chest; a CT scan of the abdomen to search for metastases in the liver and adrenal glands; an MRI of the brain to search for cancer there; and either a bone scan or a PET scan to detect any bony metastases (a PET scan is also useful for detecting cancer in other parts of the body, but not the brain). It is important to understand that wherever metastases are found, they are still composed of the same cancer cells as those found in the primary cancer. An analogy used by one of my colleagues is that an Italian who moves from Italy to the United States is still an Italian!

Another example would be that of the patient with ovarian cancer I described earlier. Although cancerous growths were found in her lungs, Alice did not have lung cancer. Instead, she had ovarian cancer that had metastasized to the lungs. The same ovarian cancer cells that were detected when her ovarian tumor was biopsied would be found in her lung tumors if they had been biopsied. For any cancer, this principle is true. Prostate cancer that has spread to the bones is not "bone cancer" but still prostate cancer, now also growing in the bones; pancreatic cancer that has spread to the liver is not "liver cancer" but the same pancreatic cancer cells that have now traveled to the liver (fig. 3).

I recently cared for a thirty-five-year-old man who came to our hospital emergency room complaining of severe back pain. Mike put off coming to the hospital because he was frightened that he would be told he had cancer, and so he delayed seeing a doctor. He worked in construction and kept blaming his symptoms on his work. By the time Mike came to the hospital, he had been suffering for months, was in excruciating pain, and was having great difficulty moving his arms, which had become numb.

On physical examination, Mike was found to have a large mass replacing his testicle. CT scans of his spine showed a tumor pressing on his spinal cord, which explained the pain, arm weakness, and numbness he was experiencing. CT scans of the rest of his body showed widespread

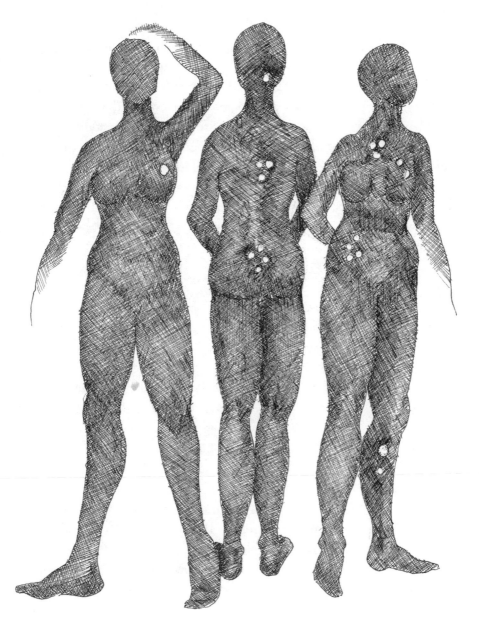

Fig. 3. *Metastasis*
When a cancer forms metastases, it spreads from the original site (pictured here in the breast) to other parts of the body. Illustration © Gale V. Parsons.

tumors throughout his lungs and in the lymph nodes of his abdomen and pelvis. The testicular mass was removed in surgery and revealed testicular cancer. Mike asked me if he needed a biopsy of the other tumors, and I told him he did not. From knowing that testicular cancer spreads by way of lymph nodes in the abdomen to the lungs and other organs, I concluded that the presentation, or entire picture, of his condition was compatible with all the masses being derived from the original cancer in his testicle. The same cells would be found in the other tumors. No further biopsies were needed. Mike received four months of strong chemotherapy treatments, and his cancer went into remission. Additional surgery was eventually needed, but the cancer is, we hope, cured.

Understanding How Cancer Spreads

The ability of a cancer cell to spread—to break away from the original tumor and grow in another location in the body—is a defining trait of cancer. In normal tissues, the cells are tightly bound and have snug "stitching" between them, like the patchwork pieces of a quilt. Benign growths, such as moles or warts on our skin, are also made up of cells that are tightly bound and cannot travel or invade the healthy tissue underneath them. For this reason, benign tumors are cured once they are removed.

Inside a cancerous growth, however, are cells that have found a way to separate from their neighbors, to loosen and dissolve the stitching that binds them. The freed cells can then be swept away by the flow of blood in a nearby blood vessel to other locations in the body. The ability of cancer to form new blood vessels is called "angiogenesis"; this property is essential for a cancer to grow beyond a very small size and to have a chance at gaining access to the circulation. Cancer cells also travel through another network of vessels, called lymphatic vessels. These channels drain our organs of excess fluid and debris and also serve as a highway on which immune cells travel throughout the body.

Once cancer cells enter the bloodstream or lymphatic channels, few of them actually form metastases (fewer than 0.1 percent of circulating cancer cells). Some are killed in the circulation, whereas others die after a period of attachment to a distant organ. Even those that do establish a home in a new location may never develop into harmful tumors. Some will enter a period of prolonged dormancy, whereas others will multiply and die at equal rates, yielding a lack of net growth. These varied fates of disseminated cancer cells help explain how some metastases can manifest themselves ten or more years after the original cancer was treated: for unknown reasons, the dormant or nonproductive cancer cells suddenly acquire the ability to duplicate themselves successfully without limit.

If metastasizing cancer cells can be thought of as the "seed," then the new environments in which they are trying to grow (most often the liver, lungs, bones, and brain) can be thought of as the "soil." The "seed versus soil" hypothesis of cancer growth was first introduced more than a hundred years ago. For the past century of cancer research, the focus has been on understanding how the seed grows, ignoring the contribution of the soil, but this is changing.

We now know that the organs to which cancer cells spread must provide growth-promoting chemicals as well as a blood supply if the cells are to grow there; similarly, plants grow better in fertile rather than barren soil. Provocative new research suggests that one person's soil may be different from another's. In other words, one person's liver may be more hospitable to cancer metastases than another person's liver. The factors that determine these differences await further discovery.

The final and most straightforward way that cancer spreads is by direct invasion of nearby tissues. A growing tumor can expand beyond the site of origin and take root in nearby structures. For example, a bladder cancer can break down the bladder wall and invade the nearby rectum; a large thyroid cancer can extend out of the thyroid and into the muscles of the neck; a lung cancer can invade an overlying rib and cause severe pain. In these situations, the cancer is said to be "locally advanced," in contrast to metastatic cancer, which is defined by distant spread in the body. The distinct ways in which locally advanced and metastatic cancers are treated is discussed in chapter 6.

There are some common misconceptions about how cancer spreads. Some people avoid undergoing operations to remove cancerous tumors because of a mistaken belief that the disease is spread through the air during surgery. And I have heard patients wonder if cutting into a tumor as part of a biopsy before its removal, or even in the more definitive surgery, can spread cancer in the body. With regard to the first belief, cancer cells cannot become airborne, nor can they survive in the air even if they were to become airborne. Certainly, if this were the case, coughing or the sharing of body fluids could spread cancer. Infections can be spread in these ways, but cancer cannot. With regard to the second concern, isolated reports of cancers tracking along biopsy routes have been reported, but this is not believed to be a significant way cancer is spread.

In sum, a cancer diagnosis represents the point of discovery of a process that began with the conversion of a healthy, controllable cell into one that can grow (multiply), spread, and survive without regulation. These properties constitute the foundation of cancer. They are central to understanding the diagnosis, behavior, and treatment of any cancer.

2
Diagnosis, Staging, Curability

I first met John when he walked into my office with his children for a consultation. He was in his sixties, of average build, with a gentle face, curly gray-black hair, and the appearance of someone whose work was physical. He wore jeans and a T-shirt with a pack of cigarettes rolled up in one side. His hands were rough, his talk straight. I would later come to know him as a happy, garrulous, backslapping man, a man's man who would do anything for his friends and family. In time, he would come to treat me as a son and endlessly philosophize about life, women, and what counted, hoping something would sink in that might do me good; sometimes I even managed to get a word in edgewise about his health.

On that day, however, John was a crushed man, for he had recently been diagnosed with advanced cancer and told that it was "terminal." Two weeks before we met, he had gone to the emergency room complaining of sudden, severe abdominal pain. A CT scan revealed multiple tumors in his abdomen and liver. Soon after, he underwent a liver biopsy, and it showed "poorly differentiated carcinoma." He met with an oncologist who told him he had, not liver cancer, but a type of cancer called "unknown primary." This diagnosis means that a cancer starts in an organ (such as the breast, pancreas, lung, or prostate) and spreads to other regions in the body but the original cancer can no longer be found (carcinoma of unknown primary is discussed in chapter 3). John was told that he had a very aggressive form of it and that his life span would be measured in months, even with treatment. To make matters worse, John felt that the doctor was matter-of-fact and offered him no hope, something he could not accept.

With his head hung down and eyes glazed red with emotion, John gave me a soft-handed shake as he sat down. He shook his head to clear away the heavy webs of grief and spoke in a steady voice. "Doc, I've come to you because I know about you. I heard you came from that big cancer center in the city, Sloan-Kettering. I know what I have is not good, but I've come to you for hope. I need someone to help me fight this battle, even if I lose the war." His devastated children nodded and touched him as if to transfer some of their strength.

It is moments like these that make me feel as though my head is in a vice. I so want to make things better. I want to be a magician, defy the reality of a bad diagnosis, and pull the proverbial rabbit from a hat. But I know the difference between wiggle room and a fait accompli. In this case, although I thought the other doctor would be correct in the end, I saw one little stone left unturned. "I spoke to the pathologist who read your biopsy. I asked him to perform additional testing on the sample, which can sometimes indicate the exact organ of origin. But he is unable do so because the sample is too small. Your first biopsy was taken under CT scan guidance. Though it may not change anything, I want you to undergo surgery so we can have a larger chunk of tumor for analysis."

I felt that if I could not help him to live for much longer, I could at least give this man what he needed right then, a true sense of hope. He needed to leave my office believing that I believed there was hope for his survival and that I would fight for it. "Doc, I know you're not a miracle worker, but I feel you'll fight for me. I'll do whatever you say if you think it can possibly help."

The operating surgeon removed the needed piece of cancer but could do little more than that because of the large masses of tumors that filled

John's abdomen and liver. Yet the surgery was worth it. The new pathology report changed the diagnosis. John did not have a carcinoma; instead, he had a rare type of sarcoma (a tumor derived from the supportive, connective tissues of the body) called GIST.

When John returned to my office with his wife, Sue, it was clear that his condition was deteriorating fast. His eyes had a sunken look, he was visibly in pain, and his belly was swollen. "John, you have a rare type of cancer called GIST, which stands for gastrointestinal stromal tumor," I said. "Our current methods of treating cancer with chemotherapy and radiation are useless against this cancer. But I have made some calls and found out that an important clinical trial at Dana Farber Cancer Institute in Boston is studying a drug called STI-571 to treat GIST. The drug is working wonders in patients with leukemia and appears very promising against GIST. I have spoken with the people in charge of the study. They're expecting you."

I walked them to the door and gave Sue two prescriptions. On one I wrote "Oxycontin," for pain. On the other I wrote "STI-571," with the contact phone number in Boston. "Don't leave Boston without it," I whispered in her ear. Sue bear-hugged me and looked me right in the eyes, speaking volumes without words; she turned away and they were gone.

One month later, John strutted into my office, and I laid eyes on a new man. "Hey, Doc, how are you? I'm great, no pain, eating again, haven't felt better in months!" He had an impish grin and twinkling blue eyes and gripped me in a strong handshake.

John was in the original group of patients who received STI-571 (later named imatinib/Gleevec) in a clinical trial that demonstrated its remarkable activity against GIST. He went on to live another two and a half very enjoyable years and touched the lives of many others.

Making a Diagnosis of Cancer

John's story illustrates many aspects of oncology, but the first is that cancer often gets diagnosed after it calls attention to itself either by causing a symptom (pain, bleeding, cough, headache, fatigue—virtually any-thing) or through an abnormal growth ("a lump"). If these are brought to a doctor's attention, tests are ordered to investigate the reason for the symptom, and a biopsy (surgical sampling) of any abnormality is performed straightaway.

The material obtained from a biopsy is analyzed by a pathologist (a physician expert at making diagnoses from the appearance of tissue under the microscope), who may make the diagnosis of cancer. Under the microscope, cancer reveals itself as cells growing in a disorganized pattern, in contrast to the organized appearance of normal tissues. In addition to diagnosing the type of cancer, the pathologist will also assign it a "grade," which relates to how aggressively it appears to be growing and how likely it is to spread. A cancer can be low, intermediate, or high grade, in order of least to most aggressive. A prominent example of how grade influences cure is in prostate cancer, in which each can-cer is assigned a Gleason score between 2 and 10. The Gleason system divides prostate cancers into those that are low grade (2–4), intermedi-ate grade (5–6), and high grade (8–10); a score of 7 can be intermediate or high grade depending on details of the pathology report. The higher the Gleason score, the lower the chances for cure after treatment with surgery or radiation.

As indicated in John's case, pathologists play a critical role in diag-nosing and interpreting cancer. Because the pathologist's impression is in part subjective and may be imprecise, it is sometimes necessary to obtain a second pathologic opinion on a biopsy sample to make certain of the diagnosis.

Cancer patients should ask their oncologists if there is any uncer-tainty in the diagnosis and whether it would be helpful (and worth the expense) to have another pathologist confirm the findings.

One of the most common ways for cancer to be detected today is during a screening test, such as a mammogram or examination of the inside of the colon by colonoscopy. Prostate cancer is screened for with palpation of the prostate gland (called a digital rectal exam) and measurement of the PSA (*prostate specific antigen*) in the blood; PSA is a protein shed by prostate cancer cells into the bloodstream. Routine screening for some cancers has been proven to save lives and is one reason that cancer death rates are declining. Screening offers the best opportunity to catch a cancer when it is at its earliest and smallest phase of growth. Current cancer screening guidelines can be found at the American Cancer Society web site, www.cancer.org.

Unfortunately, there are no effective screening tests as of yet for a number of cancers, and the disease is not often detected during a routine physical examination or blood testing. Most cancers are detected when they cause symptoms that lead a person to seek medical help.

WHEN CANCER CAUSES SYMPTOMS

More often than people realize and contrary to popular belief, a cancer diagnosis is not always a straightforward affair. Cancer may cause symptoms that develop gradually, over months, or suddenly, necessitating urgent medical attention. These symptoms may be caused by the primary tumor or by a cancer's distant metastases—tumors causing a problem in another organ (this is explained in the discussion below). Indeed, cancer declares itself in many ways, and some of them can be misleading. This is a common source of frustration and angst for patients and their primary physicians alike.

Symptoms from a cancer often mimic those caused by common ailments, so doctors first think of the more common reasons for a person to exhibit a symptom, and rightly so. (Exceptions would be if there is a strong family history of cancer that should make the physician more vigilant for signs of that cancer.) It is certainly possible that a headache may be caused by a brain tumor, but it is far more likely that there is a benign cause, such as tension or migraine. Stomach pain can be a sign of stomach cancer, but it is much more likely to be caused by an ulcer. A cough can be a sign of lung cancer, but it is far more likely to be caused by the more common ailments of a cold, postnasal drip, or asthma. If symptoms persist or worsen, further tests are performed and may uncover a cancer.

Another way cancer can masquerade is if it occurs in a person who has a chronic disorder and the symptoms are similar to those caused by that ailment. For example, a person with chronic back pain from arthritis who develops more back pain in the same region would be thought, at first, to have a worsening of arthritis. If a cancer is lurking, too, it may take time before the patient and physician realize that this pain is different and perhaps not responding to the usual remedies. If the symptoms are tolerable and the person chooses to live with them, some months may pass before further testing is performed. When the cancer is ultimately found, the patient may feel that the doctor "missed" the diagnosis earlier. But the doctor may be very skilled and diligent and treated the patient according to the likeliest situation, that the symptoms were simply a worsening of arthritis. In time, an MRI or a CT scan of the affected region would be done and reveal a tumor rather than arthritis; a biopsy would be done to diagnose cancer. It would have been impossible for the doctor to know from the outset that the new symptoms were caused by cancer.

This case illustrates the complexity of medicine and the challenges in being a physician. It also underlines the difficulty in being a patient, in conveying symptoms accurately and in monitoring (even complaining about!) a symptom that is not improving. More than any test, the patient's words, that "something is just not right," will lead the doctor to find the root of a medical problem. My perceptive mother was way ahead of her time, many years ago, when she inculcated me with this wisdom: "Listen to your patients, they will let you know what is wrong with them. They know their bodies better than anyone else."

Another way cancer can present itself is when a metastasis, rather than the primary cancer, causes symptoms. An example would be a person who develops pain in the region of the liver. A CT scan is ordered, and it shows growths in the liver that look like cancer deposits that have spread to the liver from another location (this is much more common than primary liver cancer). Because one of the more common places for this to happen is from the colon, a colonoscopy is performed. During this procedure, a tumor is found in the colon, and biopsy reveals colon cancer. Here symptoms caused by the spread of cancer ultimately led to the identification of the primary cancer. Another example of this follows next.

AN EMERGENCY DIAGNOSIS

Tom came to the emergency room of our hospital because of a sudden onset of headaches, blurred vision, and uncontrolled twitching of one of his arms. A neurologist evaluated him, diagnosed him as having a seizure, and ordered an MRI of his brain. The MRI showed numerous tumors growing in his brain that were characteristic of cancer that had spread from another location in the body. Tom was admitted to the hospital for further evaluation. Because he was a smoker, a CT scan of his chest was performed, which revealed a tumor in one of his lungs. Biopsy of the tumor revealed lung cancer, and he was diagnosed with stage IV lung cancer because of distant metastases to the brain. Tom received antiseizure medicines, steroids (medicines related to cortisone) that reduce brain swelling caused by tumors, and brain radiation. After his condition improved, he was discharged from the hospital with plans to treat the rest of his cancer as an outpatient.

Tom's story illustrates how cancer can sometimes strike suddenly and dramatically, causing a person to seek urgent medical attention. Like heart attacks and stroke, cancer emergencies require immediate treatment. Because the possibility of cancer is usually not foremost in the mind of a patient who seeks emergency care, a cancer diagnosis under these circumstances often creates tremendous stress. Martin was a forty-nine-year-old man who had been in excellent physical condition until sudden severe shortness of breath and dizziness led him to be rushed by ambulance to our hospital. A chest X-ray and CT scan showed that a large mass in the middle of his chest (in a region called the mediastinum) was impeding the flow of blood to his lungs and brain. Martin rapidly underwent biopsy of the mass, and it disclosed an aggressive lymphoma. His condition was worsening by the hour, and he needed treatment urgently. Yet he and his wife, Anne, were very analytical, highly intelligent people who wanted to know all about lymphoma and the different treatment options before they would consider treatment. Their friends also told them to get a second opinion before commencing treatment. They were not sure what to do.

For Martin's welfare, I needed to put a halt to his and Anne's indecisiveness. I told them firmly that they needed to make a leap of faith and do something extremely important: trust me. Ordinarily, I explained, I would never dissuade a cancer patient from seeking a second opinion. But in this situation, there was no time to get one at another center. It was not even safe to transfer Martin to a larger hospital, for this would unacceptably delay his treatment. Our hospital had the expertise to make him better, I said, and they needed to let us try. A second opinion could certainly be obtained once Martin was out of danger and discharged from the hospital in better condition.

This meeting was one of several between us in just two days, so Martin and Anne were ready to put their trust in me and commence treatment for his cancer. Fortunately, his lymphoma responded beautifully to chemotherapy and immune treatments, and within days of his first treatment he was feeling better. On discharge, he had a second opinion consultation that agreed with our strategy. It is now more than four years since his diagnosis, and he has been back to normal health for some time; Martin's lymphoma is, we hope, cured.

ADVICE FOR THE NEWLY DIAGNOSED

Being newly diagnosed with cancer in the hospital is one of the most difficult circumstances in which you and your loved ones can find yourselves. In Martin and Anne's case, he was sick and needed treatment before leaving the hospital. The couple wanted to trust their oncologist but weren't sure if they could or should. Yet whether you are in a hospital or at home, every newly diagnosed cancer patient faces similar immediate issues.

First, if you have suddenly become sick and the cause is cancer, you must try to come to terms with the fact that a mysterious and frightening disease is the cause of this dramatic change of health, rather than a more familiar, non-life-threatening condition. Second, you must consider accepting complicated therapies, such as chemotherapy or radiation, that may cause significant side effects. And you and your family have to make decisions about which oncologist and which cancer center to place your trust in. If you need hospitalization, you may need to rely on a new hospital and new health care providers whom you did not seek out in the first place.

All cancer patients should feel confidence in their oncologist, surgeon, and radiation therapist as well as the center in which they will receive treatment. Since this confidence is something that must be deserved and earned, however, you should try to evaluate if the hospital and physicians have the expertise and capability to treat your type of cancer. This usually means asking about the training and experience of the doctors, the reputation and accreditation of the hospital for the treatment of cancer, and whether the hospital has a research program that provides access to clinical trials. Outpatients who are not experiencing any symptoms from cancer have more time to make these decisions.

> *Great cancer care involves far more than surgery, radiation, and the administration of chemotherapy. Caregivers must always consider the totality of a patient and how cancer will impact his or her life and loved ones.*

Oncology nurses, family therapists, spiritual advisers, and other professionals should be available to assist the oncologist in addressing the many emotional and psychological needs of a cancer patient and his or her family members. Although these needs may seem secondary in the whirlwind of trying to figure out how best to save a life, it is actually at these times that you can take the measure of a cancer program: Are you and your loved ones being supported with information, education, and caring professionals who have the time to guide you through this difficult moment in your life? The answer should be yes. It takes a community of dedicated professionals to care for a cancer patient. This care should be delivered in a pleasant, warm, and welcoming environment. If the right care can be delivered near one's home or work, then that is the optimal situation.

If you are hospitalized and do not feel that the facility you are in is expert enough in your type of cancer, you should inquire about the feasibility of being transferred to a more specialized center. An outpatient can more easily seek other opinions elsewhere. Above all, if you have cancer, you should be made to feel that your oncologist is your advocate and that he or she will tell you where the most appropriate place is for the treatment of your cancer, whether this is a regional hospital or another facility. In the words of the acclaimed journalist Marjorie Williams, who wrote of her battle with liver cancer in the book *The Woman at the Washington Zoo,* "There is nothing like having a doctor who really cares about you." Amen to that!

SECURING THE DIAGNOSIS

Just as important as making a proper diagnosis of cancer when it exists is not making the diagnosis prematurely without definitive proof. Although this point may seem obvious, the reality is that medicine can be complex. Pathology results are sometimes not definitive, biopsies may need to be repeated, and a sample may need to be evaluated by several expert pathologists before a correct diagnosis is rendered. A guiding principle in the practice of oncology is that, with rare exception, absolute proof of a cancer diagnosis must exist before any treatment is initiated. Sometimes the biopsy needs to be sent to outside consultants who require additional time, so a definitive diagnosis may not be obtained for a week or more. Most patients understandably become anxious and upset when they are told, "We still don't know exactly what type of cancer you have, but we are performing more sophisticated testing, which will take more time." Yet because of how important it is to be correct, and the fact that the entire treatment plan follows from the diagnosis, this time spent waiting is worth the wait.

Janet was referred to me after having been told that she had multiple myeloma, a bone marrow cancer. She walked into the examination room quietly in visible pain owing to a recent fracture of a spine bone. Her face was downcast but showed a mixture of physical discomfort and fear. Janet was helped onto the examination table by her husband, Dave, who stood erect and imposing, right beside her. She let him do most of the talking. He was tough looking. With a fierce gaze, he stared unblinkingly at me as he spoke in short, strong phrases. "This is my baby, she saved my life when I was down," he said, as he got choked up and brought her snugly to his chest with his arm. "Now it's your job to save her life. I know you won't fail us. I won't let it happen." A shiver ran down my spine. I told them I would do my best to make her well, because I fight for all my patients as if they were my family. I quickly focused on her situation.

Janet was thought to have multiple myeloma after an abnormal protein was found in her blood and a biopsy of the fractured vertebra showed some of the cells that are typically found in that bone marrow cancer (myeloma is discussed in chapter 3). But I was not convinced by the whole picture. I ordered an additional analysis of the cells, and it showed that they were not cancerous but rather were part of the body's normal immune reaction to injury. Further investigation for myeloma cells in other parts of her body failed to turn up any sign of the disease. In the end, Janet was spared a cancer diagnosis and remains without evidence of myeloma five years later. Her pain was adequately addressed, her condition improved greatly, and she and her husband were grateful. I was extremely happy for them and breathed a sigh of relief for myself.

Because of the enormous weight placed on pathology results, I highly recommend that every cancer patient make certain that his or her oncologist is satisfied with the findings and diagnosis of the pathologist. If there is any uncertainty, have the specimen reviewed by a pathology consultant at another hospital.

Determining the Extent or Stage of Cancer

Once a cancer diagnosis is made, the next step is to determine whether the cancer has spread from its site of origin and, if it has, to locate all the places in the body where it is growing. The process of accomplishing this is called the "staging workup," because after it is completed, the cancer will be assigned a "stage." The stage is extremely important to know because treatment plans are designed based on the extent and location of the cancer. The stage of a cancer directly correlates with the likelihood of cure: in general, the higher the stage number, the more widespread the cancer and less favorable the outcome.

It is important to realize, however, that the relation between stage and prognosis is not absolute. Some stage I cancers can behave aggressively and return to take the patient's life, whereas some stage IV cancers can be eradicated. Several factors in addition to stage affect the survivability of a cancer (these are discussed below, in the section titled "Estimating Curability").

The staging workup typically involves the following: (1) imaging studies, such as X-rays, CT and MRI scans, bone scans, and sometimes PET scans, all of which locate cancer throughout the body (other kinds of testing may also be required, as dictated by the type and location of the cancer); (2) analysis of surgical results, especially if a cancer and its nearby lymph nodes are removed—in this case, the pathologist will be able to assign a "pathologic stage"; and (3) blood tests to measure tumor markers (see the table in chapter 1) and how well the bone marrow, kidneys, and liver are functioning.

The staging system for the most common cancers (such as breast, lung, and colon cancers) recognizes that there is a direct relation between the extent of cancers and their ultimate curability. The extent of a cancer is described by the TNM staging system, in which *T* stands for the size or extent of the primary *T*umor (fig. 4), *N* stands for the number and location of lymph *N*odes that contain cancer (fig. 5), and *M* stands for the presence or absence of distant *M*etastases.

T1　　　　　　　　　　　T2

T3　　　　　　　　　　　T4

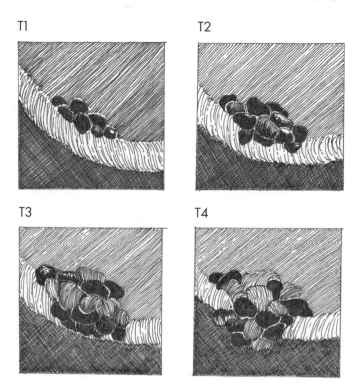

Fig. 4. *The tumor (T) staging of cancer*
The deeper a cancer grows into the tissues beneath it, the higher the T stage.
Illustration © Gale V. Parsons.

Each cancer is staged according to its own TNM classification system. Once a cancer receives T, N, and M assignments, the three elements are combined to define the stage, which commonly has four categories: I, II, III, or IV. For example:

◆ A one-and-a-half-centimeter (half-inch) breast cancer primary tumor (T = 1) that has not spread to axillary lymph nodes (N = 0) or other parts of the body (M = 0) would be stage I based on a T1, N0, M0 designation. By contrast, a one-centimeter (one-third-inch) tumor (T = 1) that has spread to five axillary lymph nodes (N = 2) but nowhere else in the body (M = 0), would be stage III (T1, N2, M0).

N0   N1

N2   N3

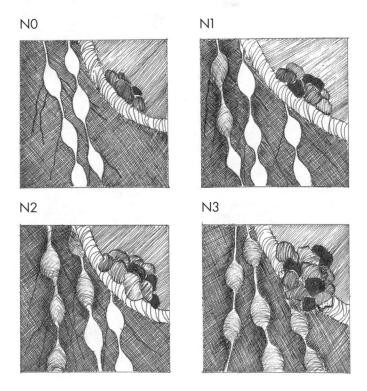

Fig. 5. *The node (N) staging of cancer*
The more lymph nodes that harbor cancer, the higher the N stage. Illustration
© Gale V. Parsons.

- A T1 lung cancer measuring three centimeters (a little over an inch)
  or less that does not involve lymph nodes would be stage I (T1, N0,
  M0); if the cancer has spread to nearby lung lymph nodes, it would be
  stage II (T1, N1, M0); if it has spread farther to involve lymph nodes
  in the middle of the chest (mediastinum), it would be stage III (T1,
  N2 or N3, M0).
- In pancreatic cancer, the stage is determined mainly by the size and
  extent of the tumor rather than whether there is lymph node involvement. For example, cancers that extend beyond the pancreas but *not
  into* nearby arteries would be classified as T3, stage II, whereas cancers that *do* involve major arteries are classified as T4, stage III. In
  general, surgeons will be able to remove a stage II cancer but not

a stage III cancer. (Sometimes chemotherapy and radiation can be given first to shrink the cancer and make surgery possible; see the management of "locally advanced" cancers in chapter 6.)

Your oncologist will explain how your cancer's TNM stage was determined.

It is important to understand that although cancer *tends* to spread first to nearby lymph nodes and then to more distant sites in the body, it does not always follow such an orderly or obvious path. A person may be diagnosed with an early-stage cancer, not involving any lymph nodes, and still develop stage IV disease years later. The explanation for this is that cancer cells either bypassed the lymph nodes and spread through the bloodstream or did pass through the lymph nodes but left no traces behind. Researchers are developing methods based on the genetic profile of a cancer that will enable oncologists to predict more accurately which early cancers have the potential to return and which can be cured by surgical removal alone.

In general, the lower the stage, the better the chances are that a cancer can be cured. Yet the fact that cancer relapses affect some individuals with low stages of cancer forms the basis for administering cancer treatments even after surgery has removed all visible evidence of the disease. Such "adjuvant" therapy is discussed in depth in chapter 6.

The TNM staging system does not apply to cancers of the brain or to the blood and lymph cancers leukemia, lymphoma, and multiple myeloma. These cancers have their own unique staging systems because they behave very differently from the more common cancers. For example, in leukemia, the cancer cells circulate in the bloodstream throughout the body; they would all be metastatic under the TNM system. In fact, most leukemias are not staged but are instead "classified" by the specific genetic defects they harbor. Multiple myeloma, Hodgkin lymphoma, and non-Hodgkin's lymphoma do have established staging systems. To learn more about the staging of blood cancers, visit the web sites listed in appendix 2.

Estimating Curability

The first thing that some patients (or their loved ones) think when they are told that they have cancer is that they might die soon. This is natural. In fact, few people die of cancer soon after they are diagnosed, although rapidly fatal cancers can occur. More people are living longer with cancer than ever before, and a cornucopia of new drugs being tested today offers real hope to cancer patients. Statistics on all persons diagnosed with cancer in the United States from 1990 to 1999 indicate that 63 percent survived at least five years (many are presumed cured). Still, not enough people do survive cancer for long enough, and we cannot escape the present-day reality that cancer claims far too many lives. Therefore, the first question that many (but not all) people with cancer ask of their oncologists is, "What is the prognosis?"

In considering the prognosis, you and your oncologist should address two central questions: First, is there a reasonable expectation for cure? And second, if the cancer is not considered curable, what is the estimated survival?

It is vital for patients and their loved ones to have a clear understanding of whether the cancer they are confronting is likely to be cured. Some cancers are cured with surgery or radiation alone; others require chemotherapy; still others, such as the blood and lymph cancers, may require a stem-cell transplant to achieve cure. If the cancer is potentially curable, then you will need to discuss the recommended treatments, their side effects, and how treatment will affect all facets of your life.

If cure is not a likely possibility, then you will need to discuss all of the above plus another crucial element: the goals of treatment. Is long-term disease control a realistic goal? Is short-term comfort and relief of suffering a more appropriate objective? Will a goal intermediate between these two be more achievable? The treatment of curable cancers and those not likely to be cured are discussed in chapter 6.

The type of cancer, stage of the cancer, medical condition of the patient, and the effectiveness of available treatments are critical determinants of a cancer's curability. Oncologists weigh these plus a number of other factors in estimating prognosis (these are discussed below, in the section titled "The Five Elements of Prognosis"). Before we explore how doctors estimate prognosis, it is important to understand what is meant by "incurable cancer."

UNDERSTANDING INCURABLE CANCERS:
EVERY PATIENT IS UNIQUE

As might be expected of all good accountants, Mitch W. walked into my office, greeted me cordially, sat down, opened a notebook, took pen in hand, and prepared to discuss "the facts." The facts, however, were not a client's tax returns but rather Mitch's returns after meeting with a renowned surgeon in search of a radical cure for his newly diagnosed cancer.

One month before our meeting, Mitch developed sudden abdominal pain and turned yellow, the sign of jaundice, indicating trouble in the flow of bile through the bile ducts. He was admitted to our hospital, where testing showed gallstones both in his gallbladder and lodged in the common bile duct, the main river of bile flow. Gastroenterologists relieved the obstruction in the duct with a stent, and he was soon off for routine surgery to remove his gallbladder. Immediately on viewing the gallbladder, however, the surgeon could tell that it was very abnormal. Frozen section (pathology done on the spot in the operating room) showed cancer. Suspicious areas in the liver and in nearby lymph nodes showed the same. The gallbladder was removed, but Mitch awoke to devastating news.

"You should have this information—the scans, pathology report, and recent surgeon's notes," he told me. "The place was huge, impressive. The surgeon was a very nice fellow. They ran some extra tests but turned me down for an operation." He stopped for a few moments, then resumed. "The cancer's too extensive. He gave me six months and told me that I should get my affairs in order. He also said that I should find an oncologist and try some chemotherapy." He successfully choked back the emotions welling up inside him and continued. "Well, my affairs have always been in order. So, here I am. I must tell you that I feel great, just took my boat out for four days . . . I'm having a very hard time believing I won't be here in six months. What do you think?"

Sometimes I think to myself in these situations, "Why am I here? Who could receive such a penetrating gaze from a fellow human?" In this case my first thought was, "How can a person be so strong, so calm in the face of his own mortality? Why should this exceptional person or anyone for that matter have to confront a deadly cancer?" But as usual, I had no answers to my questions and had to focus on the person who sought my help; I was to propose a battle plan with very inadequate weapons to combat this enemy. Mitch's strength made my job easier, and I was grateful for that. "I agree with you that six months seems grim. The average survival for stage IV gallbladder cancer is on the order of twelve months, and some patients can live substantially longer. A lot will depend on the aggressiveness of the cancer and how it responds to treatment."

Mitch began chemotherapy with a drug called gemcitabine (Gemzar), and his cancer responded surprisingly well. An MRI showed that the liver metastases were shrinking; a tumor marker named CA 19-9, measured from a blood sample, declined from 5,000 to 200 (the lower the better, normal is less than 35). After a year of nearly weekly chemotherapy treatments, he was able to stop them and enter a period of observation; his cancer was detectable but not growing. Unfortunately, soon afterward, his CA 19-9 level began to climb. Although he continued to feel well, he had to endure the mental grind of the "rising marker" (see below), first to 400, then 600, and eventually to 1,400. When it reached that level, Mitch looked at me with his head bent down, eyes peering over his glasses, and said, "Maybe it's time to get back to chemo."

During his visits, we talked about his health, our lives, and the lives of our loved ones. The physicians' offices at our cancer center are decorated with the pictures of our families, so patients become familiar with the lives of their oncologists. By this time, Mitch and I had come to know each other's body language and facial expressions. I knew he was no longer comfortable waiting.

He began a different chemotherapy concoction, capecitabine (Xeloda) and oxaliplatin (referred to as Xelox). Miraculously (to me!), the marker began to fall, reaching the 100 range; MRI confirmed the evolving remission. After eight months of treatment, his hands and feet were becoming uncomfortably numb, so therapy was halted. Still, Mitch was ever pleasant, rolling with the tides of his cancer as any good sailor would.

Not surprisingly, however, the CA 19-9 began to rise as soon as therapy ceased. Over the course of a year without treatment, while under close monitoring of his symptoms and the status of his cancer by CT scans and MRIs, the marker rose to over 10,000. He squirmed in his chair with each visit, huffed and smiled, and said, "Now what?"

To me, he seemed too well for such a high marker, even though the scans suggested that the cancer was slowly worsening. "Why don't we just start in again?" I asked myself. The truth was, I didn't know what we would use to treat his cancer, because there are no reports of third-line (or second-line, for that matter) regimens for this disease. We were in uncharted territory. I recommended that we find an appropriate clinical trial for him, testing an investigational anticancer drug; he preferred to pursue that at a later time. He appeared so well and I had such reluctance to submit him again to the side effects of chemotherapy that I recommended surgery just to prove that what we were seeing on the scans was active cancer. It did; my foray into "magical thinking" flopped. During this time, Mitch never lost his composure, never lost his sense of gratitude, never stopped boating, working, or helping other people. And he has never stopped being an inspiration to me and all those who know him.

Eventually, weight loss and other mild symptoms began to creep in and force my hand. We went back to gemcitabine and added Tarceva, a pill that is FDA approved for pancreatic cancer but has modest benefits in the eyes of most oncologists for that related cancer. Again to my amazement, the marker began to fall precipitously, back into the low hundreds. After he underwent an MRI of the abdomen, I received a call from the radiologist, which is never a good thing. "Dr. Klein's on the phone, he wants to talk to you about Mr. W's MRI," said my medical assistant, Tammy. "Oh, great," I thought to myself with trepidation, "I really don't want to take this call!"

"Rich, what's going on with Mr. W?" asked Dr. Klein.

My heart was pounding as I replied, "Where are you going with this? How can you be calling me with bad news? His marker is down and he feels well." I was not being an "objective" physician; I wanted to will a certain result from his mouth.

"That's what I wanted to know," he said. "The cancer looks much better. How is this possible?"

"I really don't know," I said, "but you made my day!"

Amazingly, Mitch has survived five years and is still going strong. To be honest, patients like him keep us oncologists going.

Rising markers. *A "rising marker" refers to the situation when a blood tumor marker (see the table in chapter 1) rises on serial measurements in the absence of evidence of a cancer relapse (as assessed by CT scans or other imaging tests) and the patient has no new symptoms that might be caused by the cancer. This situation is most commonly encountered in prostate cancer, in which a rising PSA level may be detected years after surgery or radiation, and in ovarian cancer, in which a rising CA-125 level may be detected some time after surgery and chemotherapy treatments.*

If a rising tumor marker is detected, a recurrence of cancer is not a certainty. Furthermore, if a recurrence is destined to occur, it may take years (for prostate cancer) or months (for ovarian cancer) to declare itself. Whether to institute treatment based on the rising marker alone or to wait for clear evidence of a cancer recurrence depends on many factors. These include the aggressiveness of the cancer, the patient's health, and the effectiveness and possible side effects of treatment options. For example, it is not uncommon to institute radiation or hormone therapy for a rising PSA in patients with a history of prostate cancer, but it is not common practice to reinstitute chemotherapy for a rising CA-125 in a patient with a history of ovarian cancer.

> *A rising tumor marker can create great anxiety over the prospect of a cancer recurrence. Establishing a regular schedule of doctor visits, blood draws to check the tumor marker, and surveillance testing to detect a possible recurrence at its earliest time can reduce this anxiety.*

It is, of course, devastating to learn that you or a loved one has a cancer that is not considered curable. Yet such a diagnosis does not mean that the cancer is not treatable (it nearly always is) or that the affected person may not live for many years, as in the case of Mitch. On the other hand, "six months" can sometimes be even less than that in the face of a relentless cancer that proves resistant to all known treatments.

Everyone reacts differently when diagnosed with a cancer that is not likely to be cured. Some people want to hear all the facts so that they can prepare for all possible outcomes. Others may not want to discuss the prognosis immediately and would rather wait for a time that enables them to face their situation or steel themselves to begin treatment; for some, coping means taking one step at a time. Still others do not want to talk about prognosis or hear bad news at all. Each patient's wish must be respected.

When talking with a patient who has just been diagnosed with a cancer that carries a poor prognosis, the oncologist's goal is *not* to be brutally honest, to "give" someone a certain amount of time to live, or to take away hope. Rather, the point is to get the doctor, patient, and family "on the same page," understanding the reality of the situation but maintaining enough hope and optimism to strive for the best possible outcome.

Patients should be able to convey to their caregivers their feelings, fears, and needs (physical, practical, and emotional). They should, in time, come to believe that that their oncologist will fight tooth and nail for their survival and quality of life. Every means necessary should be employed to cope with this difficult situation. Psychiatrists, social workers, family therapists, nurses, spiritual advisers, and other professionals play critical roles in helping patients and their loved ones adjust to their new reality. If these caring professionals don't come to you, seek them out!

FACING THE UNKNOWN

Many oncologists, like myself, feel a tremendous emotional burden when they have to convey to another human being that they have an incurable illness (never could I have imagined earlier in my life that I would regularly have to do this). This discussion is made all the more stressful when a patient insists on knowing how long he or she will survive.

The reason that this is so difficult to address is that no oncologist can predict the course of a patient's cancer or how it will respond to treatment. Certainly, an average survival estimate can be provided for any cancer. Yet such a number is drawn from an analysis of groups of patients and must be qualified by the recognition that *every patient is unique and reacts uniquely to cancer treatments.* Patients whose cancers respond to treatment survive longer than those whose cancers fail to respond. But how a cancer will respond to treatment cannot be known before those treatments are administered.

Furthermore, at the quickening pace of drug development today, it is possible that a promising new drug may come along that extends the lives of patients with a particular cancer. For example, in the past few years alone, several new drugs have been approved for the treatment of colon cancer, such as irinotecan (Camptosar), oxaliplatin (Eloxatin), capecitabine (Xeloda), bevacizumab (Avastin), cetuximab (Erbitux), and panitumomab (Vectibix), after decades of having just one drug (5-FU) to treat the disease. In addition, innovative combinations of new drugs with older ones are being introduced yearly, with each new combination extending life even further.

For these reasons, prognosis is not easy to predict accurately and often takes time to determine. The factors that oncologists use to try to estimate prognosis are discussed next.

THE FIVE ELEMENTS OF PROGNOSIS

Five elements go into determining the behavior and survivability of a cancer. The first four are readily known, whereas the fifth is more difficult to ascertain and is of my creation (drawn from the scientific work of many others). The five prognostic elements are:

1. The type and grade of cancer
2. The stage of cancer
3. The general health of the patient
4. The "prognostic factors" of the cancer or patient
5. The biological essence of the cancer

The cancer type, grade, and stage (elements 1 and 2) go hand in hand in determining prognosis. As discussed earlier, these two elements are by far the most important in determining prognosis. A person's general health (element 3) determines how well he or she can tolerate the recommended treatments. For example, someone with an aggressive cancer who also has severe heart problems would have a difficult time tolerating strong chemotherapy or extensive surgery. The chemotherapy doses would likely have to be lowered, and the surgery would have to be limited; these facts would diminish the chances that this person could beat the cancer. In fact, some very infirm individuals may face a greater risk of dying from other medical conditions than from their cancer; it may be in their best interest not to treat the cancer in such a situation.

Age is a consideration in determining prognosis because the older the person, the harder it is for their bodies to withstand strong anticancer treatments. On the other hand, a seventy-year-old man in perfect physical condition may tolerate cancer treatments better than a forty-year-old man who has abused his body and health, so age itself is not blindly used to guide treatment recommendations.

A *prognostic factor* (element 4) represents some medical or scientific aspect of the cancer or the patient that aids in estimating prognosis. For example, a patient who has breast cancer that has spread to axillary lymph nodes would have a certain estimated prognosis based on the stage (TNM designation) of the cancer. Beyond determining the size of the primary tumor (T) and number of affected lymph nodes (N), pathologists will analyze a breast cancer specimen for the presence of a protein called Her2/neu, or "Her2" for short. If Her2 is found on the surface of the cells, the breast cancer would be further categorized as "Her2 positive." Her2's function in the cell is to stimulate the growth of the cancer: among patients with the same stage of breast cancer, those who are Her2 positive would be predicted to have a poorer prognosis than those who are Her2 negative. Fortunately, however, an anticancer drug that specifically blocks the function of Her2, called Herceptin, has greatly improved the survival of Her2 positive breast cancer patients (fig. 6).

Two other prognostic factors used in breast cancer are the estrogen receptor and progesterone receptor. The estrogen and progesterone receptors are proteins found in normal breast tissue, as well as in many breast cancers, that bind to the hormones estrogen and progesterone, respectively. Breast cancers that make these estrogen and progesterone receptors are generally less aggressive and have a better prognosis than those that do not.

As described in chapter 1, blood tumor markers that relate to cancer growth are associated with numerous cancers, and sometimes they have prognostic importance. For example, among men diagnosed with prostate cancer, the higher the PSA at diagnosis, the lower the chances for cure; in testicular cancer, the higher the blood levels of AFP (alpha-fetoprotein) and HCG (human chorionic gonadotropin), the more difficult it is to cure.

COMBINING PROGNOSTIC FACTORS

Some cancers have "prognostic models," "scoring systems," or "nomograms" in which several aspects of the cancer and patient are combined to determine the chances that the disease will return (relapse) after initial therapy. Some of the more commonly used models are for prostate cancer (Partin Tables and several others), kidney cancer (Memorial

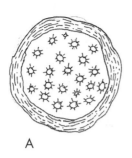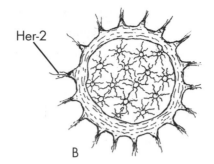

Fig. 6. *Breast cancer and Her2*
In panel A, a cancer cell is shown that lacks Her2 on its surface. In panel B, the cell contains Her2, resulting in activation of internal growth signals. Illustration © Gale V. Parsons.

Sloan-Kettering Cancer Center, or MSKCC, criteria), non-Hodgkin's lymphoma (International Prognostic Index, for diffuse large cell and follicular types), and multiple myeloma (International Scoring System).

> Helpful hint: *Ask the oncologist whether a prognostic model exists for the cancer being treated and, if so, how the cancer ranks in the model.*

Perhaps the most advanced and widely used prognostic tool has been developed for early-stage (stages I–III) cancers of the breast, colon, and lung. This tool is a computerized program called *Adjuvant! Online*, in which the oncologist enters clinical information about the patient (age and overall health) and cancer (tumor size, grade, and number of lymph nodes involved) and obtains a risk profile of that cancer. The oncologist can then choose a treatment option (such as a particular chemotherapy regimen) and the program will estimate the benefit of that treatment for the patient; the benefit relates to the reduction in the risk or chance that the cancer will return and the survival in years gained from the therapy. The results can be printed in a patient-friendly graphical format, which the oncologist can share with the patient.

The main reason oncologists want to know the risk profile or aggressiveness of a cancer is to guide treatment decisions. If a cancer is deemed to have aggressive features, then stronger treatments would be recommended to try to eradicate it and prevent it from returning; if it has less aggressive features, then strong treatments would not be necessary. This explains why cancer researchers and practitioners are so focused on identifying the behavior of a cancer before a patient starts treatment. No one wants to subject someone to strong therapies with powerful side effects if they are not truly indicated. If we can identify which cancers need strong therapies and which can be successfully treated with milder therapies, then each patient will receive the optimal and necessary treatment for his or her cancer. This is a central goal of the field of cancer medicine.

THE BIOLOGICAL ESSENCE OF A CANCER

Despite an abundance of methods to estimate prognosis, the ability to predict a cancer's behavior—to tell a patient that they will be cured if they receive treatments X, Y, and Z—is still an inexact science. This brings us to the fifth and final factor that determines prognosis. It has no official name, but I call it the *biological essence* of the cancer. It is truly the key to a cancer's behavior, even though we cannot measure it at this time. The biological essence comes from deep inside the cancer cell to dictate how heartily it grows, how well it resists apoptosis, and how invasively it spreads throughout the body. All of the properties we have discussed thus far are mere surrogates for this biological essence; they all try to approximate it but fail to truly capture it.

For example, how could it have been predicted that a fifty-year-old woman with an early-stage lung cancer (stage I) would ultimately die from lung cancer that returned more aggressively? And how could it have been predicted that a forty-two-year-old man with colon cancer that had spread to the liver and lungs (stage IV) could be cancer free five years after chemotherapy, when the average survival of such patients is under two years? Neither cancer type, stage, health of the patient, nor prognostic factors could have predicted these outcomes. These cases highlight the reality that there is much that science cannot explain about the behavior of cancer.

In scientific circles one often hears the phrase "Biology is destiny." This statement means that it is the innate biological properties, or *biological essence,* of a cancer that most strongly determines how it will behave in the body. For example, why is pancreatic cancer so difficult to treat? Its biological essence leads it to metastasize early and respond poorly to today's cancer therapies. Why is testicular cancer so often cured? Its biological essence makes it melt away with chemotherapy or radiation. When a cancer patient lives much longer than could have been anticipated, the main reason is thought to be the favorable biological essence of that cancer: it grows slower or succumbs to treatment more easily than other cancers of its class.

I have talked to enough people about cancer to learn that many know someone who defied the odds and overcame an "incurable" cancer. Certainly, in my oncology practice, I am continually amazed at how some people survive for many years with a cancer that has a dismal prognosis; the treatments worked incredibly well. But beyond the treatments, do I think that some people have a special gift, have found a cure from a healer, or have prayed harder than those who succumbed to cancer? No. I have had the immensely humbling privilege of caring for some of the most courageous, health-conscious, and devout people that anyone could ever meet; many of these individuals faced an insurmountable enemy in a cancer that just could not be beaten down. And whereas some individuals try to do all that they can to fight cancer, there are those who do not want to change their lives any more than they have to. These individuals accept the prescribed therapies but continue their life as uninterrupted as possible. This is also an important coping mechanism that must be respected. As British author and cancer patient John Diamond wrote in *Because Cowards Get Cancer Too,* "[I . . . hate] the sort of morality which says that only those who fight hard against cancer survive it or deserve to survive it—the corollary being that those who lose the fight deserved to do so."

The reality is that the biology of a cancer plays the largest role in determining why some people are cured and some are not. A person's physician and the treatments administered are clearly important; new and better cancer therapies are changing cancer's destiny in many situations. Other factors that may help a person survive include stopping smoking, eating a healthful diet, getting adequate rest and exercise, lowering stress, accepting love and emotional support, and having the will to live. But these cannot overcome an aggressive cancer for which modern medicine has no answer.

By acknowledging the reality that the molecules inside the cancer cell largely determine a cancer patient's prognosis, I do not mean to minimize the tremendous powers of the human mind, heart, and spirit. On the contrary, I would not have been compelled to write this book if I did not believe that these uniquely human traits play a vital role in the healing of the human body. Yet the cancer's biological destiny will largely determine the course it will take. Since we cannot predict this destiny for any cancer, any discussion of prognosis must be accompanied by the caveat that every person and every cancer is unique and that this uniqueness is poorly understood today.

Our ability to provide a highly accurate prognosis to a newly diagnosed cancer patient will depend on advances in science that are able to capture the biological essence of a cancer. Incredibly, these advances are happening today, and we stand at the crossroads of a new era in the field of cancer medicine. Within the next ten years, the diagnosis, estimation of prognosis, and treatments used to battle cancer will all be much more precise than they are today.

THE FUTURE OF PROGNOSIS: GENOMICS

Every person's fingerprint is unique. And so is every person's cancer fingerprint. This "cancer fingerprint" or "cancer signature" consists of all the genes a cancer is using and can be viewed as a computerized readout. Researchers are studying cancer fingerprints intensively for their ability to predict the behavior of a cancer. This field of study is called *genomics* because all the genes in a cell are collectively known as the *genome.*

To understand genomics, we need to define genes and DNA (they are also discussed in chapter 4). DNA is the genetic material that contains all the instructions a cell needs to function. But if a gene is a small portion of DNA, then a cell's genome is actually a warehouse of genes. A cell taps into only a small percentage of all the genes in the DNA warehouse at any time. Which genes the cell uses depends on its needs. For example, our skin cells can be thought of as being at rest most of the time, but if we are cut or burned, they become activated and hurl into action to repair the damage. This repair process is orchestrated by genes that were dormant but became active on injury. Thus, skin cells at rest would be drawing on a different constellation of genes than those performing repairs.

Similarly, a breast cell would use a different set of genes than a lung cell. To relate this to cancer, a breast cancer would use different genes than a lung cancer would because the two arise from different cell types. But even two breast cancers could employ different genes: a fast-growing breast cancer would use some genes that are distinct from those used by a slow-growing breast cancer (genes that direct the cell to grow fast would be more highly used in the fast-growing cancer). One can continue this line of thought down to the individual. Since no two people are alike, in personality or in DNA, no two cancers are genetically identical. Each cancer retains the genetic uniqueness of the affected person. This genetic uniqueness or cancer signature can be captured and measured on a "gene chip" that is the size of a dime.

Cancer signatures are revolutionizing cancer research and will soon drastically improve our ability to estimate prognosis for each patient and tailor specific treatments to that patient's cancer. So it merits repeating. We can rapidly analyze the many thousands of genes that exist in any cancer today. This incredible technology is enabling researchers to classify cancers by their genetic signatures and to determine which signatures portend a good prognosis and which indicate a significant chance that a cancer will return. Cancer signatures are also being developed to help guide the best and most effective treatment choices for any cancer.

For example, a one-centimeter (one-third-inch) breast cancer with cancer signature A may be easily cured with surgery, whereas a one-centimeter (one-third-inch) breast cancer with signature B may have a high likelihood of causing a future cancer relapse if treated only with surgery and radiation. The first clinically approved genomics test, called Oncotype DX, helps oncologists estimate the chances that an early stage, invasive breast cancer will relapse in another part of the body (form metastases) as well as which patients would benefit most from chemotherapy.

Breast cancers that do not involve axillary lymph nodes and that make the estrogen receptor or progesterone receptor are eligible for Oncotype DX testing. By probing the activity of twenty-one genes in a breast cancer specimen (obtained from a small piece of the stored remainder of the original surgical specimen), a "recurrence score" is generated that places the cancer in a low risk (6.8 percent), intermediate risk (14.3 percent), or high risk (30.5 percent) of developing distant metastases within ten years.

The recurrence score is also used to guide the choice of therapy, as follows: those in the low-risk range derive little benefit from chemotherapy and would typically be treated only with hormone therapy (such as tamoxifen or an aromatose inhibitor, see chapter 7), whereas those in the high-risk category derive great benefit from chemotherapy (a 28 percent reduction in the risk of a cancer recurrence at ten years). There is uncertainty, however, about how best to treat those with an intermediate risk score, which is why this group of patients is the subject of an ongoing clinical trial called TAILORx. In this study, patients with intermediate recurrence scores are randomized (randomly chosen by a computer) to receive either hormone therapy or chemotherapy plus hormone therapy. The goal is to determine whether chemotherapy prevents a cancer recurrence and improves survival compared to hormone therapy alone in this group of breast cancer patients.

Gene-based tests like Oncotype DX are being developed for nearly every type of cancer, with cancers of the lung, colon, and prostate furthest along. The future of cancer diagnosis will increasingly operate like this: the pathologist will make the diagnosis, and the medical oncologist or surgeon will order genomics testing of the specimen to help determine both prognosis and the optimal treatment for that cancer. The hope is that genomics testing will allow us to tailor cancer treatments specifically to each individual case.

3

Understanding Specific Cancers

Donna, a forty-five-year-old teacher, feels a lump in her breast. She has surgery to remove the mass, and the pathology shows a lymphoma. Donna is surprised and asks, "Do I have breast cancer?" The answer is no, she has lymphoma of the breast, not breast cancer. Her staging workup, treatment options, and prognosis will follow the principles established for lymphoma, not those for breast cancer. She will not have to undergo more surgery to test the lymph nodes in the armpit for cancer in a procedure termed axillary lymph node dissection; she will not need a bone scan to check for metastatic cancer affecting the bones. These might have been done had Donna been diagnosed with breast cancer. Instead, she will undergo CT scans of the chest, abdomen, and pelvis, lymphoma-directed blood work, a bone marrow biopsy, and possibly a PET scan to stage the lymphoma fully and plan for its treatment.

I bring Donna's case up to illustrate that many kinds of cancer can arise from the same location in the body. The type of cancer that develops depends on the specific cell type affected by the cancer process. Because every organ and gland in our body is made up of a variety of cell types, several kinds of cancer can occur in any region. For most sites in the body, one type of cell is usually affected, resulting in the common types of cancer that are most often talked about. For example, breast cancer arises from the cells of the breast glands and is more specifically described in a pathology report as "breast carcinoma." When less commonly affected cells are struck by cancer, then one of the rarer cancers occurs, such as a lymphoma or sarcoma of the breast. These principles will become clearer in the paragraphs that follow.

Although there are hundreds of distinct types of cancer, I group them here into four main categories for ease of understanding:

1. Carcinomas
2. Hematologic malignancies (blood and lymph cancers)
3. Sarcomas
4. Brain tumors

I encourage you to read about each type of cancer even though you may be interested in just one kind. The more you know about cancers and their properties, the better you will understand the specific cancer(s) you may encounter.

Carcinomas

Every organ in the human body is made up of a mixture of cells that cooperate to support the functions of that organ. For example, the heart contains cardiac muscle cells that enable it to pump and nerve cells that transmit electrical signals that spark the muscle to pump in a rhythmic fashion. Another example is the breast or mammary gland, whose main function is the production of milk to sustain the newborn. Breast milk is produced by the glandular portions of the breast, composed of glandular (or gland) cells. The gland cells are surrounded by fatty tissue, which is made up of fat cells. The glands and fat are given structural support by fibrous tissue and are supplied with blood and nutrients by arteries, veins, and lymphatic vessels. All of these parts of the breast except for the glands can be viewed as supporting elements and are collectively referred to as "connective tissue." In addition, lymph nodes containing immune cells are present in the breast, just as they are throughout the body (fig. 7).

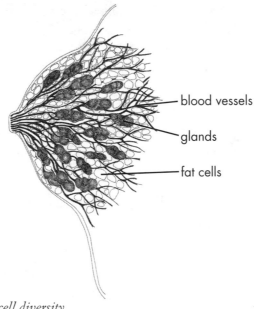

blood vessels

glands

fat cells

Fig. 7. *Normal cell diversity*
The diversity of cells that is present in each of our organs is represented here
by the normal structure of the breast. Illustration © Gale V. Parsons.

The glands of the breast are composed of a branching system of ducts
and lobules surrounded by fat. These glands react to the levels of female
hormones circulating in the body. As levels of estrogen and progesterone fluctuate during the menstrual cycle, the breast glands swell and
shrink. During pregnancy, a tremendous increase in the level of estrogen stimulates the growth and expansion of the ducts and lobules, cul-
minating in milk production (lactation). Therefore, the cells that line the
ducts and lobules of the breast glands are dynamic and strongly affected
by their hormonal environment. This fact will become relevant when I
discuss the effects of hormones on the growth of breast cancer.

The glandular cells of the breast are derived from a type of cell called
an epithelial cell. Epithelial cells tend to pack closely together to form
a continuous layer of cells called the epithelium, which forms the inner
and outer linings of many body surfaces. The epithelium protects the
tissues beneath it from the outside world. In addition to the breast, other

tissues that contain epithelium include: skin, where it is better known as epidermis; the inner lining of the gastrointestinal tract, which consists of the mouth, throat, esophagus, stomach, small intestine, and colon; the liver, pancreas, and gallbladder; the lining of the lungs and bronchial tubes; the kidneys, ureters, bladder, and prostate gland; and the uterus, fallopian tubes, and ovaries. The epithelium is also responsible for the release of important products, such as digestive enzymes made by the pancreas that enable us to absorb the nutrients in food.

Whether it is a hot sun burning the skin, spicy food wreaking havoc on the stomach, or cigarette smoke singeing the throat, the epithelium is our first defense against the elements. As such, there is considerable wear and tear on the epithelium and the need for injured and old cells to be replaced with new ones; many new skin cells are created every day as old ones are sloughed off. This high rate of cell turnover, coupled with the direct exposure of epithelium to environmental toxins, places it at increased risk for being damaged and converted into cancer.

Cancers derived from epithelial cells are called carcinomas. Carcinomas account for most of the commonly occurring cancers in adults. In contrast, carcinomas occur only rarely in children (leukemia, lymphoma, and brain tumors account for half of childhood cancers). The ten leading cancer sites for adult men and women are listed below in order of decreasing frequency.

The most common cancer sites for men are:

1. Prostate
2. Lung
3. Colon/rectum
4. Bladder
5. *Non-Hodgkin's lymphoma*
6. *Melanoma*
7. Kidney
8. Oral cavity and throat
9. *Leukemia*
10. Pancreas

The most common cancer sites for women are:

1. Breast
2. Lung
3. Colon/rectum
4. Uterus
5. *Non-Hodgkin's lymphoma*
6. Thyroid
7. *Melanoma*
8. Ovary
9. Kidney
10. *Leukemia*

Those cancers that are not carcinomas are indicated in italics. Lymphoma and leukemia arise from blood or lymph-forming cells rather than epithelial cells. Melanoma, in contrast to other skin cancers that are carcinomas (basal cell and squamous carcinomas), derives from distinct cells called melanocytes rather than epithelial cells.

Although ten cancers are listed here, the top three for men (prostate, lung, and colon cancers) and women (breast, lung, and colon cancers) account for more than half of all cancers. Many other less frequently occurring cancers are also carcinomas, such as testicular cancer and cancers of the larynx (voice box), esophagus, stomach, anus, liver, gallbladder, and sweat glands.

It follows then, that a person diagnosed with a cancer at one of the above sites can look at his or her pathology report and see the word "carcinoma." This means that the pathologist can tell from the appearance of the cancer under the microscope that it originated in an epithelial cell in the affected site. Therefore, most patients with ovarian cancer have "ovarian carcinoma," those with colon cancer have "colon carcinoma," those with prostate cancer have "prostate carcinoma," and so on. Many are also labeled "adenocarcinoma," the most common form of carcinoma. I didn't say that *all* patients with these cancers have carcinoma, because other kinds of rare tumors can affect these sites. The devil is in the details; patients affected by rare tumor types are made aware of the differences by their oncologists.

Within each broad category of carcinoma there are many subtypes, classified by pathologists based on variations in how they appear under the microscope. For example, carcinomas of the lung can be of the small cell (15 percent of cases) or non-small variety (85 percent of cases). The non-small cell tumors can be further classified as squamous cell carcinoma, adenocarcinoma, large cell carcinoma, and other types. In the case of breast cancer, although ductal carcinoma is the most common type, some other varieties include lobular, inflammatory, medullary, and tubular. The pathologic classification of cancer is anything but simple! The specific subtype of a carcinoma is noted in pathology reports.

If you are a cancer patient, the specific subtype of carcinoma that you are dealing with may be important to know because rarer forms of common cancers may follow a different course or be treated differently than the more common forms. For example, tubular carcinoma of the breast tends to be less aggressive than the more common invasive ductal type and may not require chemotherapy. Similarly, knowledge of lung carcinoma subtypes is important because targeted drug therapies may work best on particular subtypes of lung cancer: the drugs Iressa and Tarceva appear to work best against the bronchioloalveolar subtype of non-small cell lung cancer. Every patient should review the key findings of the pathology reports with his or her oncologist.

CARCINOMA IN-SITU

Thus far, we have been considering carcinomas as cancers that pose a threat to life because they are "invasive," which means that they have the potential to metastasize to other parts of the body. A pathologist will usually include the term "invasive" or "infiltrating" in a pathology report to indicate this important aspect of the cancer. For example, a tumor of the larynx may show "invasive squamous cell carcinoma," one from the stomach, "invasive adenocarcinoma," or one from the breast, "infiltrating ductal carcinoma." The terms "invasive" or "infiltrating" will be used when the pathologist sees the cancer cells invading through the first tissue barrier underneath it.

The term "invasive" in a pathology report does not mean that a cancer has metastasized, only that it might have done so.

If a tumor biopsy shows invasive carcinoma, then a staging workup (see chapter 2) will be undertaken to determine if any cancer deposits can be found elsewhere in the body. This evaluation is often performed before surgical removal of the primary tumor but in certain cases may be performed afterward. The results of the staging workup determine the "extent of the disease" and whether surgery can remove or has removed all visible areas of involvement.

Not all carcinomas, however, are invasive. One class of carcinoma is considered "pre-invasive." This type of cancer is called carcinoma in-situ (Latin for "in site" or "in place"). Under the microscope, carcinoma in-situ (CIS) does not penetrate the tissue barriers beneath it. Although CIS cells are growing in the characteristic disorganized way that identifies the tumor as a cancer, they have not yet acquired the ability to metastasize—to break into surrounding tissues and gain access to the blood or lymph stream to spread to other parts of the body. CIS does not pose an imminent threat to life, but it can develop into invasive carcinoma over time and must be treated. Most cases of CIS are surgically removed if detected, rendering the patient cured of the CIS and eliminating the possibility that invasive cancer will develop from that area of carcinoma in-situ. CIS is not treated with chemotherapy, but radiation and hormonal therapy may play a role in treatment, especially in breast cancer. The cure rate for CIS is almost 100 percent.

In addition to being an "early cancer" that is highly curable, carcinoma in-situ is also an indicator that the affected person is at an increased risk for the future development of cancer (both in-situ and invasive types). Therefore, after someone is treated for CIS, he or she should undergo regular surveillance testing to detect newly developing cancers at their earliest, most curable stages. In addition, CIS marks an important moment in the health of a patient: it is an ideal time to take advantage of cancer prevention measures or make lifestyle changes (related to smoking, diet, and exercise, discussed in later chapters) that help ward off the disease.

Carcinoma in-situ is most commonly encountered in the breast. The detection of ductal carcinoma in-situ (DCIS) of the breast has dramatically increased since mammography has replaced simple physical examination as the primary way in which breast cancer is detected today. Mammography enables the detection of much smaller cancers than are found by physical examination alone, and an increasing number of these smaller cancers consist of DCIS rather than invasive breast cancer. Many women who develop DCIS are advised to take the drug tamoxifen for five years after DCIS is treated in order to prevent the future development of breast cancer. Tamoxifen blocks the stimulating effects of estrogen on breast cells and reduces the future occurrence of both DCIS and invasive breast cancer. These cancer-reducing effects are experienced by both breasts, not just the one in which the DCIS is found.

Carcinoma in-situ is found in other parts of the body much more often than is widely recognized, in part because patients are usually told that they have, not CIS, but rather "a tumor that is the step before [invasive] cancer." For example, CIS can be found in a bladder polyp that may call attention to itself by causing blood in the urine. To screen for cervical cancer, a Pap smear is performed, which may lead to a diagnosis of dysplasia or cervical intraepithelial neoplasia (CIN); the most severe form of dysplasia is CIN III, which is equivalent to carcinoma in situ. Other areas in which CIS can be found include the colon, prostate, thyroid, oral cavity, testicle, anus, and lung. Interestingly, both carcinoma in-situ and invasive cancer are sometimes found in the same tumor, indicating that the invasive cancer grew out of the CIS. This stepwise development of cancer is discussed in chapter 5.

CARCINOMA OF UNKNOWN PRIMARY SITE

Imagine being told that you have cancer in one or several regions of your body but that the doctors cannot determine where it started. In other words, you have metastatic cancer without a corresponding primary tumor to indicate where the cancer began. The liver, bones, lungs, lymph nodes, or other areas may be affected but in a way that indicates that the cancer spread to them from some other primary location. Investigation of the breast, prostate, lungs, gastrointestinal tract, and other organs, however, fails to reveal the tumor of origin.

People who have this perplexing and frightening condition frequently request that a total body CT scan be performed in an effort to locate the primary tumor. Often, however, a full-body CT scan, an MRI, and even a PET scan cannot locate the primary cancer. Patients may seek numerous opinions and go to the biggest cancer hospitals in the hope that some doctor will be smart enough to figure out where the cancer began. These efforts are natural and thoroughly understandable. In the end, however, neither a sophisticated test nor the most skilled physician will be able to uncover the cancer source. The diagnosis will remain carcinoma of unknown primary site (CUP).

Carcinoma of unknown primary site is not on the list of the most common cancers. I have yet to hear it mentioned in the news, and I have never met a new patient who was familiar with it. One would think it is a rare type of cancer. Yet surprisingly, CUP accounts for approximately 5 percent of cancers, making it a disease that oncologists are quite familiar with. This type of carcinoma has been the subject of many clinical trials and has been studied by cancer researchers for many years. There are standardized ways of treating it in all its manifestations.

Patients with CUP must suffer the anguish of battling a cancer they cannot understand and cannot easily describe. Most tell others that they have "bone cancer," "liver cancer," or another type depending on where the disease is most burdensome; to describe CUP invites questions and doubts about the diagnosis. Some CUP patients I care for ask me at nearly every office visit to explain their cancer again and to review once more where it could possibly have come from. CUP is not only an enormously frustrating cancer but also a lethal one, with average survivals of less than two years.

Most cases of CUP are thought to represent the metastases of a carcinoma that either completely shrank away (involuted) or is too small to be detected by current methods. Pathologists will perform numerous tests on the cancer specimen to try to determine its origin. When such tests fail to identify an organ of origin, the diagnosis is CUP. It is hoped that sophisticated genetic analyses of CUP tumors will yield more accurate ways of classifying them; these tests are undergoing validation in clinical trials.

Cancers of unknown primary site are usually treated with chemotherapy and sometimes also with radiation therapy. Some patients can be cured if the cancer is localized and not disseminated in the body, in which case surgery may play a role. Better treatments are clearly needed for advanced cases of CUP. Researchers are trying to gain a better understanding of how CUP develops so that greater strides can be made against this cancer.

Blood and Lymph Cancers

The blood and lymph cancers, also called hematologic malignancies (*hema* is Greek for blood), are a complicated group of diseases that are related by their common origin in cells that comprise the blood and lymph systems of the body. All blood and lymph cells are born in the bone marrow. Some remain there, some circulate in the bloodstream, and others populate the lymph tissues found throughout the body, most prominently the lymph nodes and spleen. There are three major categories of hematologic malignancies:

1. Leukemia
2. Lymphoma
3. Multiple myeloma

Because these cancers grow in the bone marrow and/or the lymph nodes and spleen, they cause alterations of blood counts, enlargement of lymph nodes, or defects in the body's immune defenses, resulting in infections. Any one of these changes may prompt an evaluation that leads to the diagnosis of leukemia, lymphoma, or myeloma. Unlike many carcinomas, these cancers cannot be screened for or caught at a preventable stage because their natural growth patterns lead them to be present in many locations in the body at the time of detection. For example, leukemia and myeloma affect the bone marrow (throughout the body), and lymphomas often affect different lymph node regions in the body. Because of this, they nearly always require treatments that travel throughout the body—namely, drug therapies.

Surgery plays a minor role in managing blood and lymph cancers. Radiation therapy may be used in conjunction with drug therapies, depending on the clinical situation: a patient with a large mass of Hodgkin or non-Hodgkin's lymphoma in the chest, for example, is usually treated with chemotherapy followed by radiation therapy, resulting in a very high cure rate. Isolated tumors of multiple myeloma (called plasmacytomas) may be treated with radiation. Leukemia is not treated with radiation except as part of a stem cell transplant procedure, when it is given to the whole body in an effort to eradicate the disease. These examples do not encompass the full spectrum of radiation use in these cancers.

The care of a patient with a hematologic malignancy is usually managed by a physician trained in both oncology and hematology. Advances in treating these cancers are occurring rapidly, and many new promising drugs are being developed each year that require testing in clinical trials. Hematologists/oncologists in the community and those in large cancer centers often work together to plan a treatment strategy for their patients, which may include a stem cell transplant or participation in a research trial testing new medicines.

Despite their similarities, each of these three disorders is distinct. Each arises from a different type of bone marrow cell, grows differently in the body, causes different symptoms, requires specific treatments, and has varied rates of curability. In order to gain an appreciation for the blood cancers, it is helpful to have a working knowledge of how normal blood and lymph cells are produced in the body.

BONE MARROW STEM CELLS GIVE
RISE TO ALL BLOOD CELLS

When I refer to blood cells, I mean the white blood cells, red blood cells, and platelets that circulate in the bloodstream and do the work of the blood system. Their levels are routinely measured by a blood test called a CBC (complete blood count). White blood cells are part of our immune system and protect us against infection; red blood cells carry oxygen throughout the body and maintain our energy; platelets enable blood to clot. Under normal circumstances, there is one main kind of circulating red cell and one kind of platelet, but there are several types of white blood cells. The two most important are neutrophils, which help us fight bacterial infections such as "strep" throat, caused by a bacterium called streptococcus; and lymphocytes, which attack viruses, produce antibodies against infectious agents, and create a memory bank of past infections that is rapidly activated on reinfection with the same bug (this is an example of "immunity"). There are two main types of lymphocytes, T-cells and B-cells. The "T" or "B" designation relates to whether the cell matures in a special lymph gland in the chest, called the thymus (T-cells), or in the bone marrow (B-cells). Like B-cells, T-cells are born in the bone marrow, but they migrate to the thymus, where they develop further.

The bone marrow is so named because it is found inside our bones, in a place called the marrow cavity. Nearly all bones contain bone marrow. Bones are constructed of a thick outer shell, called the cortex, that has been likened to ivory and can support the weight of our bodies. Inside the cortex, in the marrow cavity, the bone thins out in a fine lacework that is filled with a spongy mixture of fibers and cells called stroma. The stroma provides a nutrient-rich, nestlike environment on which the blood cells develop and is critical to their growth.

Another word for stroma is "microenvironment." Stroma exists in every organ and represents the source of blood and nutrients that all cells, including cancer cells, need in that location. The bone marrow stroma supports the growth of all cancers that grow there, whether they are the hematologic malignancies that originate from bone marrow cells or other types of cancer that metastasize to the marrow; metastatic cancers of the prostate, breast, lung, and kidney frequently involve the bone and bone marrow.

My reasons for introducing concepts such as stroma and microenvironment are not purely educational. New cancer therapies targeting the stroma, rather than the cancer, are now being used to treat cancer patients. Three prominent examples include: (1) angiogenesis inhibitors, a class of drugs that blocks the blood supply to tumors; (2) bisphosphonates (Aredia and Zometa are examples), medicines that block the ability of cancers growing in bone to cause fractures by altering the bone environment; and (3) the related drugs thalidomide (Thalomid) and lenalidomide (Revlimid), which are effective treatments for multiple myeloma in part because they disrupt the connections between myeloma cells and the surrounding bone marrow stroma.

The bone marrow is the most active organ in the body, churning out billions of blood cells daily. Amazingly, all the different mature blood cells derive from a mother cell, called a bone marrow stem cell. These stem cells are continuously renewing themselves and maintaining normal levels of mature blood cells at all times; when necessary, they increase blood cell production. For example, during anemia, when the red blood cell count falls below normal levels, the stem cells make more red cells. And when a bacterial infection strikes the body, the stem cells ramp up production of white blood cells to fend off the invader (leading to an elevation in the white blood cell count on a CBC).

The hormone that stimulates stem cells to produce red blood cells has been made into a drug marketed under several names, including erythropoietin (Procrit, Epogen) and darbopoietin (Aranesp). These drugs improve the anemia and fatigue caused by kidney failure and chemotherapy and help avoid the need for blood transfusions. New concerns about the safety of these medicines have limited their use. When used according to guidelines established by experts in the field, however, these medicines are safe and helpful.

Similarly, the molecules that the body produces to stimulate stem cells to make white blood cells have been made into drugs, called filgrastim (Neupogen), sargramostatin (Leukine), and pegfilgrastim (Neulasta). These medicines have greatly improved the ability of cancer patients to fight and prevent infections and receive chemotherapy at the recommended intervals in order to treat their cancer optimally. A medicine that helps raise platelet counts, called oprelveken (Neumega), is also available. New drugs that stimulate the bone marrow are in development.

White blood cells, red blood cells, and platelets are the final products of a complex biological process that converts an immature stem cell into these mature blood elements. Many types of cells are formed along the pathway leading from stem cell to mature cells, resulting in the wonderful diversity of cells that one sees in a normal bone marrow biopsy specimen. In a blood or lymph cancer, this diversity is replaced by a monotonous population of cancer cells, such as the blast cells of acute leukemia or plasma cells of myeloma (fig. 8). The result is a fall in normal blood production and low blood counts, leading to many of the symptoms experienced by patients with leukemia, myeloma, and certain lymphomas.

To diagnose a blood cancer, a bone marrow biopsy is performed as part of the initial workup. Although leukemia and myeloma always affect the bone marrow to some extent, lymphoma does not always do so. In addition to pathologic analysis of the specimen, a small amount of liquid marrow may be sent for specialized testing. These tests include:

1. Chromosome analysis and molecular testing to determine if the chromosomes of the cancer cells have been altered or if genetic abnormalities associated with specific diseases can be identified. For example, if a physician suspects that a patient has chronic myelogenous leukemia, the presence of a gene called Bcr/Abl in the marrow confirms the disease.
2. Flow cytometry, a procedure in which the cancer cells are passed through a sophisticated machine called a cytometer that determines the specific molecules present on their outer surface. This procedure

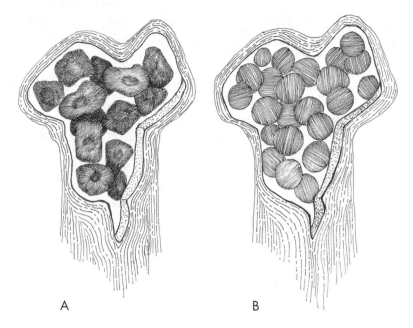

A   B

Fig. 8. *Normal diversity versus cancer monotony*
In panel A, a diversity of cell sizes and shapes is shown to comprise the
normal bone marrow. In panel B, normal bone marrow diversity is replaced
by monotony, the overgrowth of one type of cell, the cancer cell. This occurs
wherever cancer grows. Illustration © Gale V. Parsons.

can determine, for example, if a lymphoma is of B-cell or T-cell origin
and whether it contains a protein called CD20, which is the target of
several effective antibody treatments for lymphoma (Rituxan, Zevalin, and Bexxar).

In the following sections I discuss some of the hematologic malignancies with a focus on their unique features and how advances in cancer
research have greatly improved their management.

LEUKEMIA

Leukemia refers to a group of cancers in which the malignant cells circulate in the bloodstream: the word "leukemia" derives from the joining of two Greek terms, *leukos,* or "white," and *-emia,* meaning "of the

blood." Because blood cells are created in the bone marrow, the marrow is always involved in cases of leukemia. There have been tremendous advances in our understanding of the scientific basis of leukemia. Thousands of genetic changes that are critical to leukemia development have been documented, and probably more is known about the science of leukemia than about any other cancer. This knowledge has recently begun to pay off in dramatic improvements in treatment, especially for chronic myelogenous leukemia.

I have found that when a person is first referred to me with an abnormal blood count, the disease he or she fears most is leukemia. This is because most people think of leukemia as being a rapidly fatal disease. The truth is that although some types of leukemia can indeed be rapidly fatal if not treated successfully, others may not need to be treated for twenty years or more.

There are four main types of leukemia: acute myelogenous leukemia (AML), acute lymphoblastic leukemia (ALL), chronic myelogenous leukemia (CML), and chronic lymphocytic leukemia (CLL). Acute leukemias (AML and ALL) usually need to be treated soon after diagnosis, whereas chronic leukemias usually do not need urgent treatment because they grow more slowly, often do not cause symptoms, and may remain stable without therapy for months or, in the case of CLL, several years. Leukemia can be treated with chemotherapy, more specific targeted therapies, stem cell transplantation, or a combination of these approaches. Space limitations prevent a discussion of each type, so I focus here on CML, a disease that has become the model for the future treatment of all cancers, and on CLL, the most common type of leukemia.

CHRONIC MYELOGENOUS LEUKEMIA

Chronic myelogenous leukemia is characterized by an initial slow-growing phase, followed three to five years later by an aggressive and uniformly lethal phase (if not treated). Fortunately, we know more about CML than about any other cancer. In fact, CML is a disease of firsts. It was the first disease to be labeled "leukaemia," in 1845 by the famous German pathologist Rudolf Virchow, who described several patients with elevated levels of "colorless corpuscles" (representing white blood cells) and enlarged spleens. In what marks a turning point in cancer research, CML was the first cancer to be associated with a specific chromosomal abnormality, termed the Philadelphia chromosome, after the city in which the discovery was made; this established, for the first time, that cancer is marked by alterations to DNA. Most recently, CML came to be the first cancer to be treated with startling success by a new wave of cancer treatments called targeted therapies.

CML arises when a bone marrow stem cell experiences a genetic mutation that results in the exchange of genetic material between two chromosomes. As a result, a gene called Bcr becomes joined to another gene called Abl. The resulting Bcr/Abl fusion gene gives rise to a powerful mutant protein that makes the cell grow faster, resist cell death, and acquire the characteristics of a leukemia cell. Bcr/Abl is essential for the development of CML; the discovery of ways to inhibit its function has revolutionized the treatment of this disease.

For many years the only hope for cure of CML was a bone marrow transplant from another person. In 1999 a drug called imatinib (Gleevec) was approved by the FDA based on extremely positive results in the first stages of testing. Gleevec is a pill that is well tolerated by patients and specifically shuts down the action of Bcr/Abl. CML cells die when Bcr/Abl stops functioning, and many patients achieve a complete remission of their disease.

It is too early to tell if Gleevec is curing CML permanently, but the drug has enabled many patients to delay, if not completely avoid, the need for bone marrow transplantation. Remarkably, for those patients in whom CML grows after an initial response to Gleevec, new drugs such as dasatinib (Sprycel) and nilotinib (Tasigna) are effective in reestablishing remission in many cases. It is hoped that CML will remain a disease of firsts and become the first leukemia to be cured by medicines that work with pinpoint accuracy rather than with intensive chemotherapy or transplantation.

CHRONIC LYMPHOCYTIC LEUKEMIA

Unlike the three other types of leukemia, the cell of origin in CLL is not the bone marrow stem cell but rather a mature lymphocyte (lymph cell). This cell does not have the innate explosive growth capacity of a stem cell or the ability to form any cell other than another lymphocyte. These differences account, in part, for the less aggressive course of CLL in comparison to the other leukemias. CLL is often diagnosed when routine blood testing reveals an elevated white blood cell count and all other laboratory tests are normal. The abnormal lymphocytes of CLL may reach very high levels in the bloodstream without causing ill effects.

CLL is the most common form of inherited leukemia, although the vast majority of cases do not run in families. Patients with a family history of CLL may wish to help researchers discover the genes responsible for this inheritance pattern by donating a sample of blood. They can ask their oncologist or a genetics counselor for the name of a center that is researching familial CLL (see the resources listed in appendix 2).

Like other leukemias, CLL cells are found in the circulation and bone marrow. Unlike the others, however, CLL is also typically found in the spleen and lymph nodes. CLL is staged in the United States according to the Rai Classification, which segregates patients into low-, intermediate-, and high-risk groups. All patients have an elevation of the lymphocyte count (called lymphocytosis). Low-risk CLL includes stage 0 (lymphocytosis only); intermediate-risk disease includes stage I (enlarged lymph nodes) and stage II (enlarged liver or spleen); high-risk CLL includes stage III (anemia) and stage IV (low platelet count). The higher the risk category, the greater the need for treatment.

The growth of CLL in lymph nodes is very similar to the pattern of growth of lymphomas. Indeed, oncologists think of CLL more as a lymphoma than a leukemia, and it is treated most successfully with the same chemotherapy drugs and antibody treatments used to treat lymphoma. Although the treatment of CLL improves every year, the only known way to cure CLL is with a stem cell transplant from another individual. However, because CLL mainly affects older individuals and this procedure is risky, only a small percentage of CLL patients are suitable candidates for it. For any patient, treatment recommendations are based on the stage of the disease, the patient's health, and estimates of the aggressiveness of the CLL, which varies from patient to patient.

I recently met a seventy-four-year-old man in excellent health who was referred to me after he was incidentally noted to have an elevation of the lymphocyte count on routine blood testing by his primary care physician. Doug was a retired businessman who played tennis six days a week and worked around the house on the seventh day. He had never felt physically better in his life. I could tell from looking at a slide of his blood under the microscope that the leukemia cells in his circulation were characteristic of CLL. Specialized testing of the blood with flow cytometry would later confirm the diagnosis (a bone marrow biopsy is not essential to make the diagnosis of CLL).

Because he felt so well, Doug was understandably dumbfounded when I told him he had leukemia. As is often the case in CLL, however, certain features of his disease indicated that he would not likely need any treatment for many years. Instead, he would see me four times a year to monitor the disease, a policy called observation or "watch and wait" (also called "watch and worry" by some patients).

In contrast, I also care for Susan, a forty-five-year-old woman who required treatment with two chemotherapy drugs (Fludara and Cytoxan) plus an immune therapy (Rituxan) for CLL that had grown to the point that the lymph nodes in her neck were bulging visibly and her energy was declining. After one course of treatment, her lymph nodes could no longer be felt. She continued to work throughout her six courses of treatment and is now back to having the CLL merely observed. Susan will ultimately require additional treatments when the disease returns, but it cannot be predicted when this will occur.

These two cases illustrate the range of behaviors of CLL. To some, CLL is a problem only in name; it will not shorten their life span. To others, it is a life-threatening cancer. To help predict the future behavior of each newly diagnosed case, oncologists often test the CLL cells (which can be obtained from the blood or bone marrow) in several ways. These include:

1. Analysis of the chromosomes of the CLL cells; some abnormalities portend an indolent or slow course, whereas others predict a more aggressive course.
2. Assessment (by flow cytometry) of whether the cells possess two markers, ZAP-70 and CD-38. CLL that contains both markers tends to be more aggressive, whereas CLL that contains neither marker tends to be the least aggressive; the presence of one marker predicts an intermediate aggressiveness.
3. Determination of the status of a segment of CLL DNA called IgV_H (pronounced I, G, V, H). IgV_H status is either "mutated" or "non-mutated"; the mutated group carries the more favorable prognosis.

MYELODYSPLASTIC SYNDROME

Myelodysplastic sydrome (MDS) is a disorder in which the bone marrow stops being able to produce enough blood cells. It is caused by acquired (that is, not inherited) genetic damage to the marrow stem cells and mainly affects those over age sixty. The reason for the stem cell damage is usually unknown, although some cases are caused by exposure to benzene, radiation, or certain types of chemotherapy.

Analysis of the name "myelodysplasia" is the first step toward understanding this confusing disorder: *myelo* is Greek for marrow, *dys-* means abnormal, and *-plasia* means formation or development. Thus, myelo-dys-plasia means abnormal bone marrow development. The result is insufficient blood formation for the needs of the body.

MDS is usually diagnosed when weakness, infection, or bleeding causes a person to seek medical help; some cases are found on routine blood testing before symptoms arise. Analysis of the CBC will show reductions in one, two, or three of the blood counts (red, white, platelets). The patient will then be referred to a hematologist, who will rule out other causes of low blood counts (such as deficiencies of vitamin B12, folic acid, and iron) and perform a bone marrow biopsy.

A curious finding in MDS is that, although the disorder is characterized by lower than normal blood counts, a patient's bone marrow will often exhibit an excess of blood-producing cells compared to normal. The appearance of the MDS marrow cells, however, is bizarre; they are misshapen, abnormally enlarged, and altered in a way that enables them to be labeled "dysplastic." The problem is that the exuberant growth is exceeded by accelerated cell death: instead of releasing healthy blood cells into the circulation, MDS cells mostly die in the bone marrow.

Although MDS is not a cancer, the dysplastic and damaged marrow stem cells are primed to sustain further damage and be converted into leukemia. The likelihood of conversion to leukemia can be predicted with some accuracy and is highly correlated with overall survival (the greater the chance of leukemia, the lower the survival). The method of prediction is called the International Prognostic Scoring System (IPSS). The IPSS uses three criteria to determine if a patient has a low, intermediate, or high risk of developing leukemia. They are:

1. The percentage of bone marrow cells that are leukemia blasts (ranging from less than 5 percent to 20 percent).
2. The chromosome pattern of the bone marrow cells.
3. The number of blood counts (one, two, or three) that are low, considering the red cells, white cells, and platelets.

An MDS patient's hematologist will calculate the IPSS score and risk category, which will dictate the possible treatments. Those with low or low to intermediate scores may need only a low-intensity approach to maintain their blood counts, such as blood transfusions or injections of blood cell growth factors. Those with intermediate to high IPSS scores may require chemotherapy followed by a stem cell transplant from another person in an effort to eradicate the diseased marrow. Patients with any score may benefit from the drug azacytidine (Vidaza), which is a form of low-intensity chemotherapy. When Vidaza works well, it can diminish the need for blood transfusions, delay the onset of leukemia, and extend life. The related drug decitabine (Dacogen) was recently approved by the FDA for use in MDS patients with high or intermediate IPSS categories. Some patients may benefit from infusions of anti-thymocyte globulin (ATG), a horse or rabbit serum that suppresses the immune system (which may be attacking the bone marrow).

A special category of MDS is that characterized by a 5q minus chromosome abnormality (also called deletion 5q). Patients with such an abnormality in their bone marrow may respond well to the drug lena-lidomide (Revlimid), which can induce dramatic improvements in red blood counts and liberate them from blood transfusions.

LYMPHOMA

In 1832 a distinguished English physician named Thomas Hodgkin reported on a group of patients who had a rapidly fatal disease characterized by greatly enlarged lymph nodes and swelling of the liver and spleen. He did not know what caused the disease and did not mention cancer in his seminal publication. He treated one patient with "cascarilla and soda" without effect and recommended "caustic potash" for less advanced cases. Please don't ask me what these treatments were! Let's just be relieved and grateful to the physicians and scientists who have contributed to today's understanding that Hodgkin's disease is a type of lymphoma (now called Hodgkin lymphoma) and that modern treatments can cure more than 75 percent of cases.

Lymphomas are the most common hematologic malignancy. There are two main categories, Hodgkin lymphoma (HL) and non-Hodgkin's lymphoma (NHL). NHL occurs much more often than HL. The type is determined by a pathologist's analysis of a biopsy specimen. Lymphomas can arise virtually anywhere in the body because of the widespread distribution of lymph cells and lymph nodes. Although lymphomas may cause any of a number of symptoms, most cases are detected after a patient feels a swollen lymph node or the enlarged node presses on a vital organ, causing internal symptoms.

If the diagnosis is non-Hodgkin's lymphoma, testing will reveal if it derives from B- or T-cells (80 percent are from B-cells). Hodgkin lymphoma is always of B-cell origin. Current classification systems recognize five types of HL and more than thirty types of NHL. Whereas HL mainly affects young adults and those fifty-five or older, NHL typically affects those over age fifty (some forms are more common in younger individuals). In appendix 2, I list many excellent resources to learn about both HL and NHL. For the remainder of this section, I focus on non-Hodgkin's lymphoma.

Decades of sophisticated scientific research into the mysteries of the immune system have enabled us to understand the origins of the many kinds of non-Hodgkin's lymphoma. Normal lymphocytes go through a multistep process of maturation from bone marrow stem cell to fully functional infection-fighting immune cell. Each step is represented by a specific cell type, and each of these cells can be affected by the malignant process and give rise to a lymphoma. This is why there are so many types of NHL.

The oncologist will tell a patient the specific type of NHL he or she has. Follicular lymphoma and diffuse large cell lymphoma are the two most common types; less common types include small lymphocytic, mantle cell, lymphoplasmacytic (Waldenstrom's macroglobulinema), MALT (mucosa-associated lymphatic tissue), and peripheral T-cell lymphomas. The doctor will also state whether it falls into the low-, intermediate-, or high-grade category. The grade relates to how aggressively the lymphoma is likely to grow: low-grade types grow over years, whereas intermediate-grade lymphomas grow over months, and high-grade lymphomas grow even faster. To relate this to the concepts of growth and apoptosis described in chapter 1, low-grade lymphomas are marked by diminished apoptosis, whereas intermediate- and high-grade lymphomas have accelerated growth as their defining characteristic. If lymphoma can be thought of as a pot of boiling water, then low-grade lymphomas are at a gentle simmer, whereas high-grade ones are on a rapid boil.

The faster growing the lymphoma, the more urgent the need for treatment. It is also often the case that the faster growing the lymphoma, the greater the chances that it can be eradicated with chemotherapy. This is why patients with diffuse large cell lymphoma, for example, are told that there is a good chance for cure with treatment, whereas those with low-grade lymphomas are told that we do not yet know how to eradicate this disease.

As illustrated by the case of Don, the seventy-five-year-old with lymphoma described in chapter 1, some low-grade lymphomas are observed closely and not treated until necessary; approximately 20 percent will actually undergo spontaneous remission and shrink for a time without treatment. If fever, night sweats, weakness, or progressive enlargement of lymph nodes occurs, then treatment might be necessary. When the time comes, a number of highly effective treatments are available to control the disease.

Just as I have emphasized in other cancers, no two lymphomas are exactly alike. Focusing on the most common type of NHL, B-cell diffuse large cell lymphoma, about half of all cases will be cured with a treatment regimen called CHOP-Rituxan. This consists of three chemotherapy drugs administered intravenously (C = Cytoxan or cyclophosphamide, H = hydroxy-daunorubicin or doxorubicin/Adriamycin, and O = Oncovin or vincristine); an oral steroid medicine, called prednisone (P); and a genetically engineered antibody that specifically attacks B-cell lymphomas, called rituximab (Rituxan), which is administered intravenously along with chemotherapy.

Can it be predicted who will and who won't be cured with CHOP-Rituxan? Oncologists employ a prognostic system called the IPI (International Prognostic Index) to each case of diffuse large cell lymphoma to classify it into a low-, intermediate-, or high-risk category; the higher the risk, the lower the chances for cure. A related system called the FLIPI (Follicular Lymphoma IPI) can be applied to cases of follicular lymphoma. Both the IPI and the FLIPI use clinical information, such as the patient's age, the stage of the cancer, and the elevation (or lack thereof) of the blood marker LDH (lactate dehydrogenase). But it is not a perfect way to predict survival. A more sophisticated method based on determining the genetic makeup of the lymphoma (using a gene chip, discussed in chapter 2) is being pioneered and is hoped to be available in the near future.

Patients with NHL often confront a complex disease that has many good treatment options. New and effective therapies for lymphoma are rapidly being developed. Cure or long-term disease control should always be the goal. This may be achieved with chemotherapy drugs, antibody therapies, radioactive antibodies, or a stem cell transplant. Although innovative approaches such as lymphoma-specific vaccines were not successful in recently performed clinical trials, harnessing a patient's own immune system to control his or her lymphoma will continue to be a major focus of researchers.

MULTIPLE MYELOMA

Until approximately fifteen years ago, treatment advances in multiple myeloma stagnated. Patients had few treatment options, were powerless against its bone-eroding effects, and typically lived for two and a half years. Few ever achieved a complete remission. This situation changed with the demonstration that intensive chemotherapy given with the support of a patient's own bone marrow or peripheral blood stem cells (called an autologous transplant) could result in much better responses than ever seen before. More recently, the introduction of the drug thalidomide as an effective therapy for the disease has ignited research into the use of novel biologic agents for its treatment. As a result, multiple myeloma has been transformed into a hotbed of innovation and scientific breakthroughs that are extending the lives of many patients to beyond five years and some to more than ten years.

The culprit cell in myeloma is the plasma cell. Plasma cells are normal constituents of our immune system and reside mainly in the bone marrow, where they make up less than 5 percent of marrow cells. Their job is to generate antibodies, which are infection-fighting proteins that each plasma cell crafts to "form-fit" the target of its attack (for example, bacteria that cause infections). Every person's blood contains a large variety of antibodies, each directed at a specific target.

Just as any cancer arises from one aberrant cell, myeloma is caused by one plasma cell that acquires the necessary genetic mutations to become a cancer. This one cell multiplies to form many more plasma cells. Because all the plasma cells in myeloma are replicas (clones) of the first cancerous plasma cell, they all produce the same antibody molecule. This antibody is present in high enough amounts to be distinguished from all the other types of antibodies. It is detected in the blood and/or urine by a test called electrophoresis.

The antibody molecule found in myeloma is usually detected in the blood and is referred to as an M-protein (M stands for monoclonal, or one type of protein). Fragments of the M-protein, called light chains, may also be found in the urine in some patients, where they are called Bence Jones protein, after the renowned British physician Henry Bence Jones, who reported their discovery in 1847. A new test, called the free-lite assay, can detect light chains in the blood with great sensitivity and is being increasingly used to both diagnose the disease and follow its course after treatment.

A physician may order an electrophoresis test that leads to the detection of an M-protein for many reasons. These include unexplained anemia, a high protein level in the blood, reduced kidney function, bone pain, or numbness and tingling in the feet (called peripheral neuropathy). If an M-protein is detected, it is a sign, not a certainty, that myeloma may be present. A bone marrow biopsy is performed to look for excess plasma cells, and X-rays of all the bones (called a skeletal survey) are performed to examine them for damage caused by the disease; MRIs are often done to give a more precise picture of bone involvement. Myeloma cells create little holes in the bones called lytic lesions. All of these tests help determine the presence of myeloma, the stage of the disease, and whether treatment is necessary.

I wish to emphasize that a person found to have an M-protein does not necessarily have myeloma. In fact, one of the most common consultations I perform as a hematologist practicing in the community is the evaluation of a person whose blood tests show an M-protein but who is otherwise well. In these circumstances, it is not uncommon to have a normal skeletal survey and a normal bone marrow examination, without an excess of plasma cells. The diagnosis in these situations is a disorder termed MGUS, which stands for monoclonal gammopathy of unknown significance. This is a convoluted way of saying that an M-protein is present but everything else is normal, so the patient does not have myeloma. Because MGUS does have a 25 percent risk of progressing to a blood or lymph cancer over a thirty-year period, patients with MGUS need to have their M-protein, blood counts, and kidney function checked at least once a year.

A central question in trying to comprehend the effects of myeloma in the body is: Why do myeloma cells burrow into and destroy bone? None of the other blood cancers commonly attack our skeleton. This bizarre behavior of myeloma is explainable by the observation that myeloma cells and bone cells support each other's survival. Scientists have discovered that as cancerous plasma cells grow from the bone marrow into the hard bony cortex, they nuzzle up to bone cells called osteoclasts and stimulate them to eat away at the surrounding healthy bone. The bone cells, in turn, secrete chemicals that stimulate the growth and survival of the myeloma cells. This vicious cycle must be arrested or the result is severe bone weakening and fractures, which cause the pain and debilitation experienced by patients who are not responding to therapy.

Modern treatments for myeloma include not only those aimed at killing plasma cells but also those aimed at killing the destructive osteoclasts. Examples of osteoclast-killing drugs include pamidronate (Aredia) and zoledronic acid (Zometa). These medicines are given along with myeloma-fighting drugs because they are not sufficient to control the disease. The expanding spectrum of myeloma-fighting medicines includes chemotherapies (such as Doxil, melphalan, and Cytoxan), steroids (such as dexamethasone and prednisone), thalidomide (Thalomid), its derivative lenalidomide (Revlimid), and bortezomib (Velcade). The revival of thalidomide as a cancer therapy nearly fifty years after it was banned for causing birth defects is a remarkable story of the human spirit, science, and serendipity.

Ongoing studies are defining the best sequence and combinations of myeloma-fighting agents to use to improve the control of the disease and long-term survival. Organizations such as the Multiple Myeloma Research Foundation (www.multiplemyeloma.org) and the International Myeloma Foundation (www.myeloma.org) are fueling the accelerated pace of progress in this disease.

Sarcomas

William was an athletic, vigorous man who developed lower back discomfort. He thought, quite naturally, that it was caused by muscle strain or arthritis affecting the back, so he took anti-inflammatory drugs to ease the symptoms. The discomfort continued, however, and it worsened over several months, ultimately limiting his ability to move without pain. William then sought medical attention and, about that time, developed a hard bulge that protruded from the lower back area on the right side. An MRI showed that the mass was growing in the lower back and buttock region and had its origin in muscles that run along the lower part of the spinal column. The mass was biopsied and proved to be a sarcoma. Neither William nor his wife had ever heard of sarcoma. This is not surprising, because sarcomas account for only 1 percent of adult cancers.

Sarcomas are cancers that derive from the supporting structures of the body (*sarc* is Greek for "fleshy," and *sarc-oma* means "fleshy growth"). These supporting structures, or connective tissue, include muscle, bone, cartilage, fibrous tissue, fat, nerves, and blood and lymphatic vessels. They give form, provide support, or supply nutrients to the human body and comprise the framework on which our vital organs and glands are built. For example, besides the glandular elements, the breast contains fat, muscles, ligaments, arteries, veins, and nerves that surround and support the glands and coordinate their function (see fig. 7). Each connective tissue structure can give rise to a cancer that would be called a sarcoma, whether it occurred in the breast or another region of the body.

Physicians who treat sarcomas have divided the disease into two broad categories: those derived from bone and those derived from the soft tissues, such as fat or muscle. Osteosarcoma and Ewing's sarcoma are the two most common bone sarcomas and affect children and adolescents more commonly than adults. Soft-tissue sarcomas occur most often in the extremities and abdomen, though they can arise virtually anywhere in the body. For example, sarcomas of the breast are well described but account for less than 1 percent of breast cancers.

Sarcomas and carcinomas have important differences other than originating from different cell types. Carcinomas typically metastasize to the lymph nodes, lungs, bones, liver, or brain. In contrast, sarcomas usually spread to fewer locations: those that originate in the abdomen metastasize mainly to other parts of the abdomen, whereas extremity sarcomas spread predominantly to the lungs. Some sarcomas may become very large and infiltrate surrounding tissues, making them difficult to remove completely. This may be apparent to the surgeon during the operation or be revealed on analysis of the specimen by the pathologist.

There are more than a hundred types of sarcomas. Many of the names are long and complicated but do bear some relation to the tissue they start in. For example, liposarcomas are derived from fat cells (*lipos* is Greek for "fat"), and angiosarcomas are derived from blood or lymphatic vessels (*angos* is Greek for "vessel").

One sarcoma merits special attention because its treatment is unique among sarcomas. It is called GIST, which stands for gastrointestinal stromal tumor. GISTs are soft-tissue sarcomas that typically grow in the abdomen, most commonly in the stomach wall. Possible symptoms include pain, bleeding into the gastrointestinal tract, and abdominal swelling. GISTs that are not small and easily removed by surgery are incurable because they often spread throughout the abdomen. Before the late 1990s, GISTs were neglected cancers, considered to be rare and known to be resistant to chemotherapy and radiation therapy. No treatments could slow their growth, and survival was very limited. This situation changed dramatically with the discovery that the drug imatinib (Gleevec) could cause tumor regression in a high percentage of GIST sufferers.

The staging of sarcomas follows the TNM system, but as important as the stage is the "grade" of the tumor, because high-grade sarcomas have a much greater tendency to metastasize and limit survival compared with low-grade sarcomas. The treatment of sarcomas requires the combined input of an experienced surgeon, radiation oncologist, and medical oncologist to coordinate how surgery, radiation, or chemotherapy will be applied to lead to the best outcome. Referral to a specialized sarcoma center may be recommended. Helpful web sites include www .curesarcoma.org and those listed in appendix 2.

Brain Tumors

Brain tumors are a distinct category of cancer by virtue of their occurrence in a very separate and privileged region of the body called the central nervous system. This system is protected by a barrier of bones and membranes and is bathed in a compartment of clear, sterile liquid called spinal fluid. For this and other unknown reasons, tumors that begin in the brain do not spread to the rest of the body. In contrast, brain metastases represent the spread of cancer to the brain from a primary location elsewhere in the body.

Brain tumors are also unique in that the cells that give rise to most brain tumors exist only in the brain. For example, glial cells surround and support the nerve-firing cells of the brain (called neurons) and give rise to gliomas, the most common category of brain tumor.

As in other cancers of other parts of the body, there are many types of brain tumors; the specific type, grade, and location of the tumor determine the treatment approach and prognosis. Surgery, radiation, and chemotherapy treatments are tailored to each case and are coordinated by a team consisting of a neurosurgeon, medical or neuro-oncologist, and radiation oncologist.

Glioblastoma multiforme is the most frequently occurring brain tumor in adults. It is usually detected after a person experiences unremitting headaches, seizures, or neurological impairment. Maximal surgical removal of the tumor is usually followed by radiation therapy to the "tumor bed" in combination with administration of an oral chemotherapy drug called temozolomide (Temodar). It appears that those brain tumors that *do not* produce a protein called MGMT respond better to Temodar than those that make the protein; MGMT protects cancer cell DNA from the damaging effects of Temodar. Tumor testing for MGMT has not been standardized and therefore is not routinely available.

One of the most exciting advances in our understanding of brain tumors was recently made when scientists discovered that brain tumor stem cells, comprising less than 1 percent of all the cells in any tumor, may be responsible for perpetuating the cancer. New therapies will undoubtedly hone in on this critical cell population and could lead to major advancements in the treatment of brain tumors. Helpful web sites include www.abtf.org, www.braintumor.org, and those listed in appendix 2.

4
Why Cancer Develops

The wife of a patient of mine with lung cancer asked to speak to me in private. A wife and mother, Melissa was battling to keep her husband alive and her family intact. She was experiencing sleepless nights and needed answers to a number of burning questions. Melissa was trying to come to terms with what could have caused her husband's cancer at the early age of forty-six. He was a virile man, an outdoorsman and construction worker, the kind of person everyone likes instantly because of his easygoing manner and giving smile. He was also a three-pack-a-day cigarette smoker, having smoked from age thirteen until he quit at age thirty-nine. Melissa knew that cigarettes contributed to his cancer but wondered if the dusts he inhaled at work for many years could have also played a role. She was also concerned that lung cancer could run in families, and if so, whether her little boy would be at risk for cancer later in his life. As her strength rose above her sadness, Melissa wiped away her tears and said, "That's it. I'm sorry to burden you. But I need to know. I just need to know."

When you or someone you love is diagnosed with cancer, there is a compelling human need to know why the cancer occurred. Those affected by cancer naturally ask, "Why me?" "How did this happen?" "Why did I get cancer?" People have different opinions and beliefs about why they developed the disease. Some think they were destined to develop it because many of their relatives had cancer: "It's in the family." Some wonder if their diet was too high in sugar or fat. Others are convinced that unhealthy workplaces are at fault. Some people blame themselves for using tobacco products. And still others wonder about radiation exposures, alcohol, infections, other health problems, medications, stress, or impurities in the water we drink, food we eat, and air we breathe.

Who is right? Actually, everyone is right, but to a degree. Each cancer is caused by a unique mixture of factors that collectively resulted in its occurrence. Each factor exerted a certain pressure on the cells of the body that led to that cancer. Some cancers are caused by one strong factor that exerts tremendous force, like a knockout blow to a prizefighter. Others are caused by many factors that each exerts only minor force, like hitting a prizefighter with a hundred little jabs before finally knocking him out.

It is easier to identify the root causes of cancer when only one or two factors are at work compared with a variety of factors. Cancers that have a strong genetic basis, the "inherited cancers," are much better understood than are the "sporadic cancers," which affect those without a strong family history of cancer. The reasons for this are explored throughout this chapter.

An example of a single strong risk factor is in individuals who have a disease called FAP, or familial adenomatous polyposis. Those with FAP develop hundreds or even thousands of polyps in their colons beginning in childhood and have a nearly 100 percent chance of developing colon cancer by age fifty. They have inherited a genetic predisposition to cancer caused by an abnormality in a gene called APC that exists in their family's DNA. Those with FAP are counseled about why their genetic mutation leads to cancer and are advised that removal of the colon and rectum, when the polyps become too numerous to remove during surveillance, will save their lives; cancer can be averted. The scientific basis of this cancer is well understood, so patients can be told why the cancer developed.

On the other hand, a healthy man without a strong family history of cancer cannot be told with certainty why he developed prostate cancer. Numerous factors may have contributed to it, including a diet high in animal fat and red meat but low in fruits and vegetables; repeated infections of the prostate; older age; and an African American heritage. Prostate cancer affects more than two hundred thousand American men every year, the vast majority of them over age sixty. It strikes one in every six men, suggesting that the tendency of the prostate gland to develop areas of cancer may be a by-product of living to an advanced age. Clearly, the exact reasons why prostate cancer occurs are not well understood. There is no single gene, no toxic link where blame can be laid. Yet this is the usual situation for most cancer patients.

Most people diagnosed with cancer receive no satisfying answer to the question "Why did I get cancer?" Many agonize over the cause of their cancer and wrack their brains to figure out what could have brought it on. I tell them to go easy on themselves, for several reasons. First, most of the common cancers take decades to develop (see chapter 5); one would have to examine all their exposures over a twenty-to-thirty-year period to figure out which ones contributed to cancer. Second, no one can lead a perfect life, eat a perfect diet, or be born with perfect genes. Certainly, tobacco products, diets full of empty calories, and lifestyles lacking exercise are not optimal for human health and do contribute to cancer; indeed, a cancer diagnosis should provide a strong motivation to change these poor habits. Third, as explained above, *the vast majority of cancers occur for unknown reasons.* Even if every known, controllable risk factor was minimized, cancer might still occur. This is because cancer is a very complicated disease; there are few simple answers. It will take more time and more research to understand completely why we get cancer.

Fortunately, many brilliant people have dedicated themselves to unraveling the mysteries of cancer. In laboratories and scientific institutions around the world, our genes are being probed and our environment is being analyzed. Astounding progress has been made. Our highly sophisticated understanding of cancer today was galvanized in 1953 by the discovery of the structure of DNA as a double helix by James Watson and Francis Crick. Because cancer is ultimately a disease of DNA, a clear picture of DNA was needed before the field of cancer research could progress. Watson and Crick's seminal finding was to biology what the discovery of digital circuitry was to the development of computers. The ensuing fifty years has seen an avalanche of knowledge about how our bodies work and what goes wrong when cancer sets in. New cancer-fighting therapies are rapidly being developed based on this knowledge and are discussed in chapter 7.

Even so, we are just beginning to appreciate the intricacies of cancer's initiation in any one of us. It has become evident only in the past few years that most cancers arise through a complex interplay between our DNA and the environment in which we live.

When the environment interacts with DNA in a harmful way, DNA can become damaged. If the damage is not repaired, then DNA becomes permanently altered and is said to have undergone mutation. Over many years, numerous mutations accumulate in cells destined to become cancerous. These mutations to DNA drive cancer's development.

> *Cancer results when "good" DNA goes "bad."*

Cancer arises because a part of the normal or good DNA that we are born with is changed by mutations and becomes bad. Bad DNA imparts to a cell the properties of unlimited growth, ability to spread, and inability to die—the defining traits of cancer, discussed in chapter 1. But what causes these harmful DNA alterations to arise? Aren't the things that cause mutations in DNA the true *causes* of cancer? Indeed, they are.

Two main categories of factors determine whether DNA will undergo mutation: (1) our genetic makeup, or the DNA we are born with; and (2) our exposures, which include diet, lifestyle, and environment, or what we do to our DNA. These two factors are commonly called nature and nurture, respectively.

Cancer is no less determined by a combination of nature *and* nurture than are most other illnesses. Like so many human ailments, cancer often results from harmful interactions between our body and the environment. Diabetes, high blood pressure, and high cholesterol are common medical problems often brought on by a combination of poor dietary choices, excess body weight, and an underlying predisposition to these conditions. This interaction between nature and nurture is plainly summarized in a statement about the causes of multiple sclerosis (MS) in a medical textbook: "MS [is] likely triggered by an environmental exposure in a genetically susceptible host." In other words, some environmental stimulus can cause MS, but mainly in people whose DNA is susceptible to that stimulus. The same can be said of cancer.

It is the great hope and challenge of the next decade that cancer researchers will better identify both the environmental factors and the genes that lead to the different cancers. This chapter explores the forces that cause cancer. I also indicate how this information may benefit you if you already have cancer. The discussion begins with the focal point of cancer initiation, DNA.

Cancer and the Blueprint for Life

DNA provides the life spark for all living creatures, be they plants, molds, or humans. Called "the blueprint for life," DNA is awesome in power and graceful in design, a natural creation of breathtaking beauty and sweeping simplicity. Imbued with immense responsibilities, DNA is the keeper of our heredity and enables us to pass on family traits from one generation to the next. DNA holds the keys to understanding evolution, human development, and most human diseases.

Consider the role of DNA in human development. From the moment the egg and sperm fuse to form one cell called a fertilized egg, the DNA within that cell starts to work its magic and executes an ancient plan.

The DNA spearheads an explosive phase of growth that turns one cell into the trillions of cells that compose our bodies. At the same time, DNA guides some cells to form our lungs, others to form our fingers, and still others to form all our various parts. Imagine how one cell, too small to see without a microscope, can give rise to a brain with all its complex thoughts; a ticking heart, pumping blood throughout the body; eyes that see the world; a stomach that grinds food; and all the other tasks of which we are capable. And after we burst forth into the world, we passage through infancy, childhood, adulthood, and finally old age. All these changes, which may seem magical to us, are precisely choreographed by our DNA; they are also heavily influenced by the outside world (feed a developing fetus alcohol and normal development is drastically altered).

The magic, therefore, is in the workings of DNA. But what is DNA and how does it accomplish such amazing things? DNA is a stringy substance that resides in the inner chamber of each cell in a location called the nucleus. From this vantage point DNA sends forth its orders that direct the cell how to interact with other cells, when to multiply, and when to die. Whereas animals use their eyes and ears to communicate, DNA uses proteins to convey its messages. In order to make these proteins, DNA first generates a related compound called RNA. The flow of information from DNA to RNA and then to protein is called the "genetic code" (fig. 9).

If we were to look closely at DNA, we would see that it is composed of repeating units of four similar chemicals, called bases (or nucleotides): A for adenine, T for thymine, G for guanine, and C for cytosine. Each human cell's DNA, or genome, is composed of three billion bases, one connected to the next like pearls on a string. This string is not continuous, however, but is broken up into twenty-three separate units called chromosomes. When the bases are arranged in a particular order in the DNA, a gene is formed and a cell has the instructions it needs to make the corresponding protein. Although DNA contains the blueprint for the functioning of our bodies, the proteins do the actual work. Proteins are made up of chemicals called amino acids.

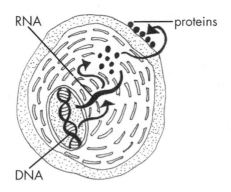

RNA

proteins

DNA

Fig. 9. *The genetic code*
DNA directs the functions of a cell by generating proteins, made through an intermediary molecule called RNA. Illustration © Gale V. Parsons.

For example, insulin is a protein that regulates blood sugar; it is made in the cells of the pancreas following the directions of the insulin gene. Similarly, red blood cells contain the oxygen-carrying molecule hemoglobin, which is made from instructions contained in the globin genes. Every gene consists of A's, T's, G's, and C's, but the specific ordering of these bases makes each gene unique. There are genes for every aspect of human functioning—from genes that control brain activity to those that make our nails grow. As they relate to cancer, there are genes that make a cell multiply and those that generate a blood supply for a growing tumor; there are even genes that can naturally antagonize these processes (hallelujah!). In total, there are about twenty-five thousand human genes as determined by the monumental accomplishment of the Human Genome Project, which deciphered all three billion bases of human DNA.

DNA UNDER ATTACK

For DNA to execute its many vital tasks properly, the genetic code must be kept pristine. But DNA is under constant attack from cancer-causing agents in the environment (called carcinogens), such as smoke, industrial wastes, food by-products, and radiation. Carcinogens cause mutations in DNA that can be as small as one base change out of three billion or as large as an entire chromosome, involving the complete loss of millions of bases. Fortunately, like the Pink Panther diamond, our cells contain highly sophisticated security systems that guard DNA and continuously probe and preen it for mutations. These systems are composed of special proteins that have as their sole charge the detection and repair of damaged DNA.

For example, sunlight contains ultraviolet radiation, which nicks and distorts the DNA strands of skin cells. And cigarette smoke releases a chemical called benzopyrene into the bloodstream, which freely passes into the body's cells to attack the DNA within. Both types of DNA damage are sensed by proteins called "gatekeepers," which bring the activities of the cell to a grinding halt and issue a command: "Repair the DNA or this cell will die!" Speeding to the scene are proteins called "caretakers," which repair damaged DNA. Caretakers grip onto the damaged region, remove the foreign chemical or injured bases, and mend the strands with healthy genetic material (fig. 10).

If the DNA sustains so much damage that the cell it directs can no longer function normally, the gatekeepers order the cell to commit suicide. In this way, our bodies are protected against the outgrowth of cancerous cells. Yet the gatekeepers and caretakers are not perfect; they cannot correct 100 percent of the damage to a person's DNA over a lifetime. Plus, they get overwhelmed: years of smoking will ultimately leave a permanent scar on DNA (and damage other cell parts), leading to such chronic diseases as emphysema and coronary artery disease or to cancer.

Although human DNA is very large (two meters, or almost seven feet, if stretched out, compacted a millionfold in the cell!), only about 1 percent of it is composed of the critical segments we call genes. The remaining 99 percent, once thought to be "junk DNA," protects and regulates access to genes and serves other functions in the cell that scientists are still uncovering. There is ample room for mutations to affect DNA without altering the integrity of our genes or the behavior of a cell. But when mutations do affect genes, the proteins arising from those altered

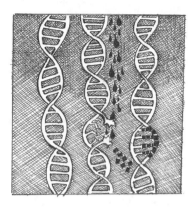

Fig. 10. *DNA damage and repair*
Normal, intact DNA (left) is shown being damaged by carcinogens
(middle) and then having been repaired by the cell (right). Illustration
© Gale V. Parsons.

genetic blueprints will be abnormal and a cell's behavior can be changed
forever.

DNA MUTATIONS ALTER A CELL'S BEHAVIOR

A cell is like a miniature factory in which each worker (protein) is responsible for carrying out a specific task for the good of the unit. Every
protein has its role. When a protein's structure is changed by gene mutation, then the function of that protein is also changed. Some mutations cause a protein's capabilities to be enhanced, like a weight lifter on
steroids, whereas others cause its role to be lost entirely.

A critical breakthrough in our understanding of cancer was the discovery by Dr. J. Michael Bishop and Dr. Harold E. Varmus that mutations in the genes that control the normal growth patterns of a cell can
transform these "good" genes into "bad" genes, which they termed oncogenes. The study of oncogenes exploded after their findings, which were
rewarded with the Nobel Prize. In contrast to normal genes, oncogenes
spawn proteins that are supercharged at promoting growth, spread, and
survival, cancer's three essential properties. These overactive molecules

are being targeted and quieted by new cancer-fighting drugs, as discussed in chapter 7.

On the other hand, mutations to genes that serve as brakes on cancer growth and survival, called tumor suppressor genes, result in the loss of these important safeguards. Gatekeeper and caretaker genes are also types of tumor suppressor genes: by repairing mutations, they prevent cancer from developing. It is much harder to replace a lost tumor suppressor gene than it is to block an overactive oncogene. Replacement requires insertion of the lost gene into cells through a technique called gene therapy, whereas blocking is accomplished with drugs. To insert a gene into every cancer cell is a daunting technical task. As of this writing, there are no approved gene therapies for fighting cancer.

The combination of generating oncogenes and crippling tumor suppressor genes leads to a toxic imbalance in the cell that tips the balance in favor of uncontrolled growth. The result of all these mutations is a full-blown cancer cell. It is thought that a minimum of four mutations are needed to generate cancer, although most cancers contain far more. For common cancers, such as prostate, breast, colon, and lung cancers, it takes many years for enough mutations to accumulate to give rise to cancer. This process is speeded up if an individual is born with a critical gene mutation, as discussed in the next section.

The dependence of our DNA on the gatekeeper and caretaker security systems to prevent mutations is made crystal clear by what happens when these systems malfunction. Their breakdown is found in nearly all cancers and is believed to be one of the earliest changes in the process of converting a normal cell into a cancerous one. We have learned a great deal about these systems from families who have a hereditary predisposition to cancer. Inherited mutations in gatekeeper or caretaker genes are common in such families.

Family Cancers

Because cancer is so prevalent, many individuals have some family history of it. These histories can vary quite a bit. One person may have only an uncle with prostate cancer, whereas another may have a brother with bone cancer, a sister with breast cancer, and a father with lymphoma. How do you know if your family medical history indicates that your family is especially prone to cancer? And to which cancers in particular? A properly taken family cancer history, genetic counseling, and appropriate genetic testing can help determine if there is a strong, moderate, or low family and individual risk of cancer (see appendix 2 for a list of helpful resources).

In trying to understand one's risk of developing cancer it is important to note that most cancers affect us in a pattern that is called sporadic: they occur in individuals without an apparent family concentration of the same type of cancer. The reasons for sporadic cancer development have more to do with environmental influences and aging (cancer is more common in those over age sixty) than to an inherited, genetic predisposition to cancer. This is not to say that one's family DNA is unimportant, because it is. What it does mean is that a single inherited abnormal gene is not the cause of most lung, colon, breast, pancreas, prostate, melanoma, lymphoma, or other common cancers.

Yet for approximately 5 to 10 percent of all those with cancer, one mutant gene, passed down in the family DNA, is the primary cause. The specific DNA mutation typically causes the corresponding protein to lose function. For example, mutations in the genes that lead to inherited forms of breast and ovarian cancer, BRCA1 and BRCA2 (BReast CAncer), prevent the full proteins from being generated; this renders them unable to perform their functions in the cell (it's like cutting off a boxer's arms). Because BRCA1 and BRCA2 function to direct the repair of damaged DNA, loss of BRCA1 or 2 activity permits a cell's DNA to accumulate the damage that can result in cancer.

Inherited genetic mutations are more widely known to cause such medical disorders as hemophilia, sickle cell anemia, Tay-Sachs disease, and muscular dystrophy. But the same principle holds for all inherited genetic diseases: a gene with an important role in the body exists in a mutant form in the affected individuals, leading to a particular health problem. In the case of muscular dystrophy, mutation of a muscle gene called dystrophin causes severe debility. In the case of family cancers, mutations are often in genes that prevent a cell from maintaining its

DNA, resulting in mutations to additional genes. These family cancer genes are called cancer susceptibility genes.

WHY DO FAMILY CANCER GENES LEAD TO CANCER?

Individuals with a family history of breast and/or ovarian cancer undergo testing of the genes BRCA1 and BRCA2 to determine if they contain mutations known to predispose to cancer. Families with Li-Fraumeni syndrome may have breast cancer, sarcomas, brain tumors, leukemias, lymphomas, and adrenal cancers; members are tested for mutation in a gene called p53.

A family history of colon cancer as well as cancers of the endometrium (uterus), ovaries, duodenum, pancreas, and kidneys/ureters, may indicate the presence of Lynch syndrome or hereditary non-polyposis colon cancer (HNPCC); the genes MLH1, MSH2, and others will be investigated for mutations.

Children who develop an eye tumor called retinoblastoma are tested for mutations in the gene Rb, the first inherited cancer gene identified.

Why do mutations in BRCA1 and 2, MLH1, p53, Rb, and other genes of this class increase the risk that cancer will develop? Because they are the caretakers and gatekeepers, DNA's security system; their normal job is to repair DNA damage, keep it mistake-free, or stop a cell from surviving if its DNA is irreparably harmed. Their absence by mutation makes DNA unstable and prone to further damage, a situation termed genomic instability. Genomic instability creates a vicious cycle of mounting DNA damage that ultimately creates numerous genetic mutations inside a cell. Although cancer is not a certainty, its risk is greatly increased. Defects in family cancer genes thus set the stage for cancer to develop. Their presence from conception accounts for the earlier age of onset of cancer in individuals who harbor them.

WHO SHOULD BE TESTED?

In general, genetic testing is recommended for those with a personal or family history indicating that a family cancer gene may be present. Some of these indicators are:

1. Cancer diagnosed before the age of fifty;
2. Multiple family members affected by cancer;
3. Two or more cancers in any individual;
4. Breast cancer diagnosed in a man;
5. The same type of cancer in a close relative (for example, sisters with breast cancer or a father and daughter with pancreatic cancer); and
6. Clustering of cancers in one family that are known to be caused by the same genetic mutation, such as breast/ovarian/pancreatic or colon/uterine/ovarian cancers.

These and other features of a family medical history are tip-offs that a family may have a hereditary predisposition to cancer. One or more members may then be asked to consider giving a blood sample so that their DNA can be tested for mutations in the specific genes associated with the types of cancer occurring in the family.

TESTING SAVES LIVES

The main reason to find a family cancer gene is to save lives. Individuals who possess the mutant gene can undergo earlier and more frequent cancer screening tests aimed at early detection, such as breast MRI and colonoscopy. Some may be advised, or elect themselves, to remove the organs at high risk in order to prevent cancer from developing.

Healthy persons at increased risk can consider taking medications to reduce their chances of developing specific cancers, such as: (1) tamoxifen and raloxifene to prevent breast cancer; and (2) finasteride to prevent prostate cancer, although it has not received FDA approval for this purpose (it is approved for the treatment of benign prostatic hypertrophy, or BPH). Women at increased risk for breast cancer and men at increased risk for prostate cancer (including all men aged fifty-five and older) should discuss the risks and benefits of taking these medications with their physicians.

If you know that you are a carrier of a family cancer gene, then you can be proactive in finding ways to prevent or better detect cancer. High-risk individuals are also encouraged to participate in clinical trials aimed at finding better ways to prevent cancer. This is a dynamic field, with new studies and recommendations coming frequently. These issues should be discussed with appropriate health care professionals, and they are described in greater length on the web sites listed in appendix 2.

On the other hand, if a family harbors a mutant cancer gene, then those members who test negative for the mutation (do not have it) can be relieved of the anxiety of believing themselves to be at high risk for cancer. They can follow routine cancer screening guidelines and would not be advised to undergo preventative surgery or other intensive measures to avoid cancer.

It is important to realize that not all families with a clear history of a family cancer will be found to have a gene mutation. This is not because the genes are not present but rather because not all the family cancer genes are known. Such families should be referred to an appropriate center that is working to identify new family cancer genes. Family members should continue high-level surveillance approaches to detect cancer as early as possible.

Getting yourself genetically tested for cancer is understandably a process fraught with emotion. There are many medical, psychological, and practical aspects to consider when performing these tests. For example, some individuals from a high-risk family avoid being tested because they fear they will be advised to have an organ removed to prevent cancer; others may feel guilty if it is discovered that they do not harbor a mutant gene but their siblings do. Some decline counseling because they fear health insurance or employment discrimination (a genetic nondiscrimination bill was signed into law in the United States in 2008). For these and many other reasons, intensive education and counseling is provided before genetic testing is performed.

> *Through a process called informed consent, all possible outcomes of genetic testing are discussed ahead of time, as are the psychological, medical, and financial ramifications of the test results.*

Your genetic counselors, physicians, family, and support systems will help you decide on the best course of action to take following the results of genetic testing. Each individual's personal preferences are always paramount.

When multiple members of a family are affected by the same type of cancer, the probability of a family cancer gene is high and the importance of the family DNA is clear. But consider the majority of cancer patients who either lack a family clustering of similar cancers or who may have several members affected by different cancers. Is their family history of any importance? Does a family's DNA influence cancer development in the commonly occurring sporadic cancers, or does cancer affect most of us randomly, without regard to our genetic constitution? Answers to these questions have only recently come to light.

Large studies of the populations of Utah, Sweden, and in particular Iceland, where nearly all cancer cases since the eighteenth century have been accurately catalogued, have shown that many cancers tend to cluster in particular families. They do not affect the population randomly. Nearly all the common cancers (on the top-ten lists in chapter 3), and even the less common cancers (such as thyroid and testicular), are found more frequently not only in the nuclear family but also in third-, fourth-, and fifth-degree relatives in some families. Even a cancer such as lung cancer affects some families more than others, separate from the effects of smoking. Moreover, a tendency to develop cancer in general (different types of cancer), rather than only one or two types, has been found in some families.

The increase in cancer risk to members of families with different types of sporadic cancers is much less than the risk associated with inherited cancer genes, such as a mutant BRCA1. Yet these findings show that one's family history is important and that a person's family DNA undoubtedly influences the development of even sporadic cancers. The specific genes that may cause family clustering of sporadic cancers are unknown at this time. An oncologist, therefore, could not recommend that genetic testing be done on individuals whose families have a variety of sporadic cancers because the tests have not yet been developed to detect the culprit genes. In contrast to the leading role played by a family cancer gene to cause a hereditary family cancer, it is believed that many different genes are each playing a "bit part" to collectively bring about a sporadic cancer. Some of these genes may be gatekeepers, others caretakers, and still others genes that help the body detoxify carcinogens in the environment. Discovering these genes is extremely important if we are to understand why most cancers develop. It is also an arduous task that will be accomplished only through painstaking and innovative research.

SUMMARY

Whether a cancer is inherited or sporadic, the types of genetic mutations that give rise to it are similar. Both types of cancers have mutations in genes important to the growth, spread, and survival of cancer. Although some mutations are inherited and give those individuals a "head start" on cancer, most occur after birth and affect the general population later in life. This is the current expert view of cancer's development and of its dependence on changes to DNA.

Cancer and the Environment

In 1981, Congress commissioned two of the most renowned cancer researchers of our time, Sir Richard Doll and Sir Richard Peto, to research the environmental causes of cancer. In their report, entitled "The Causes of Cancer: Quantitative Estimates of Avoidable Risks of Cancer in the United States Today," Doll and Peto concluded that the contributions of diet and tobacco to the development of cancer were so large that if behaviors could be changed, many cancers could be avoided altogether.

Almost thirty years and a great deal of research later, the links between poor nutritional habits and tobacco use and the development of cancer have been solidified. In addition, the promotion of certain cancers by environmental toxins (such as radiation and chemical wastes), alcohol, or infections is much better understood. Of equal importance are emerging scientific tools that clarify why some individuals get cancer from a given environmental factor, such as smoking, whereas others don't suffer the same fate.

I need to emphasize that these issues are extremely complex, involve mammoth amounts of data, and in some cases do not provide the perfect answer. This is especially true for the connection between diet and cancer: for example, the role of dietary fat as a contributor to cancer continues to be debated among experts. Although some individuals and medical "experts" feel comfortable saying that certain foods and supplements "prevent cancer" and that "the right diet can prevent 90 percent of cancers," these claims are largely unsubstantiated. I avoid such oversimplifications here and defer to the reality of the limits of our knowledge.

Although each cancer risk factor deserves its own discussion, here I focus on how diet and tobacco contribute to the formation of cancer. Following this, I describe the types of studies under way aiming to explain why the same environmental factors lead to cancer in some individuals but not in others. My goal is to clarify a few popular concepts and discuss the newest information rather than to list how diet is thought to influence each specific cancer; this information can be found in sources listed in appendix 2. For those interested in learning about the latest research findings on how food, supplements, and lifestyle impact the development of cancer, I refer you to the World Cancer Research Fund/American Institute for Cancer Research Expert Report, *Food, Nutrition, Physical Activity, and the Prevention of Cancer: A Global Perspective* (www.dietandcancerreport.org).

LIFESTYLE AND CANCER

The types of foods you eat, whether you exercise regularly, and whether you maintain a healthy body weight are major determinants of your overall physical health. Altogether, they constitute what I call a "pattern for living." Patterns for living start young; they are difficult to change in midlife; and even if they are drastically altered, healthy patterns cannot fully erase the effects of unhealthy ones.

Fortunately, I was raised to adhere to a healthy pattern for living. My mother raised us on plainly seasoned fish, chicken, baked potatoes or rice, steamed vegetables, and eggs, with an occasional steak, burger, or liver and low-fat dairy products. Food was never fried, and there were rarely any chips, sodas, or other junk food in the house. I loved to play sports and have exercised regularly throughout my forty-five years. The only smoker in my family was my father, who died at age fifty-two of a heart attack. Because of this upbringing, I rarely eat high-fat foods and have been able to maintain a stable weight. My pattern for living is deeply ingrained and I hope will yield many more years of good health (and overcome a genetic predisposition to heart disease). I will always be grateful to my mother for having the insight to know what was healthful to eat before nutrition was widely talked about. And I'll always remember her saying to me, "What are you eating that junk for?" whenever I managed to get a cookie into the house (perhaps she was a bit over the top!). This is not to say that I don't enjoy a juicy cheeseburger or a decadent hot fudge sundae, because I do—but always in moderation (once in a while).

Research has vindicated my mother's sense of which foods are healthful. A large and ever-growing number of studies indicate that cardiovascular diseases (such as heart attacks and strokes), adult-onset diabetes mellitus, and cancer are highly influenced by one's pattern for living: a diet high in red meat and animal fats and low in fruits and vegetables, obesity, and a lack of exercise constitute an unhealthy pattern for living that often leads to major illness. As I discuss below, eating the right foods, getting regular exercise, and maintaining a healthy body weight is a healthy pattern for living that optimizes your chances for a long, healthy life.

DIET AND CANCER

Diet can promote or inhibit the formation of cancer in many ways. Diet can promote cancer through: (1) the presence of carcinogens in food (which can be natural constituents or man-made additives); (2) the generation of carcinogens by cooking—for example, when foods are smoked, fried, or grilled, polycyclic hydrocarbons are produced; (3) the increased exposure of the body to carcinogens by a diet low in fiber, which slows bowel movements; and (4) "overnutrition" or excess body weight.

Some of the ways that diet prevents cancer include the ingestion of vitamins and nutrients that help our bodies detoxify carcinogens (present in cruciferous vegetables—broccoli, brussels sprouts, cauliflower, and kale) and the presence of cancer-fighting chemicals in fruits and vegetables.

In the sections that follow I discuss some of the ways in which fruits and vegetables lower cancer risk and why overnutrition increases it.

CAN FOOD PREVENT CANCER?

Trying to understand how nutrition affects cancer is difficult for a number of reasons. First, the chemistry of foods is enormously complex. Fruits and vegetables contain thousands of different compounds, called phytonutrients or phytochemicals, plus a host of vitamins, minerals, and fiber. Teasing out which plant constituents are most important for disease prevention is not easy. Second, research that involves obtaining dietary histories from individuals over many years can be inaccurate. Third, lifestyle factors other than those under study, such as exercise and changes in weight, may affect the results. For these and other reasons, we often hear conflicting reports in the news about the role of certain foods in preventing cancer. Some research is done well, some poorly; no matter, the news reports it all! No wonder people can become exasperated and lose faith in scientists to provide definite answers to important questions about nutrition and cancer.

There is ample evidence to suggest that a diet high in fruits and vegetables lowers the risk for a number of cancers. But it has been difficult to prove that adhering to a diet high in fruits and vegetables will decrease an individual's cancer risk. To try to prove the connection, researchers follow people over time and see if fewer cancers develop in those who eat more fruits and vegetables. So far these studies have failed to prove such a broad link. One explanation could be that because so many factors affect the development of cancer it may not be possible to isolate the contribution of certain foods. Another reason may be that specific types of fruits and vegetables can help particular types of people (who have a certain genetic makeup) prevent the growth of only some types of cancer. This speaks to the complexity of the interaction between our DNA and the environment, which scientists are just beginning to unravel.

Despite the lack of precise scientific guidance, there is strong evidence from the study of cancer in different populations around the world that there are both good and bad foods when it comes to influencing the development of cancer. Our Western diet, full of animal fat and refined sugars and low in fruits, vegetables, and fiber, is associated with much higher rates of breast, prostate, and colorectal cancer than a vegetarian-style Eastern diet. When people migrate from Japan and China to the United States (and other countries with similar diets), their rates of these cancers quickly rise to that of Americans, as successive generations of their descendents eat a Western rather than Eastern diet.

More direct links between particular dietary components and cancer have been confirmed by some recent studies. For example, long-term consumption of red meat and processed meats has been clearly shown to increase the chances that colorectal cancer will develop; and among more than a thousand patients treated for stage III colon cancer in a study sponsored by the National Cancer Institute, those adhering to a typical Western diet (higher intake of red meat, fat, refined grains, and desserts) had higher rates of cancer recurrences and lower survivals than those adhering to a diet high in fruits, vegetables, poultry, and fish. In postmenopausal women trying to avoid a cancer recurrence after being treated for breast cancer, the Women's Intervention Nutrition Study (WINS) suggested that a diet low in fat (15 percent of total calories) is superior to a high-fat diet. However, because the low-fat diet group also lost weight, experts currently debate whether weight loss, a low-fat diet, or both may lead to fewer breast cancer relapses. Firm dietary recommendations for breast cancer survivors must therefore await future studies.

Beyond the effect of any food or food group on the development of cancer is the increasingly important role played by being overweight or obese. This condition has been proven to raise the chances that cancer will occur. Most people know that overweight and obesity increase the risks of cardiovascular diseases and diabetes, but cancer is also on the list of diseases caused, in part, by excessive body weight. Cancers of the colon, breast (in postmenopausal women), prostate, uterus, kidney, esophagus, stomach, pancreas, gallbladder, liver, and perhaps non-Hodgkin's lymphoma and multiple myeloma are more likely to occur in overweight and obese individuals. This is of major concern because, according to cancer biologist Mel Greaves, "many of us now persistently binge, exercise too little, and live long enough for it to matter."

When it comes to following nutritional advice, I choose to be guided by the true experts. One is Dr. Walter Willett, a prominent epidemiologist and leader of the Nurses' Health Study and the Health Professionals Follow-up Study, which have rigorously recorded the diet and behavioral patterns of thousands of health professionals since the 1980s. In his book *Eat, Drink, and Be Healthy,* Willett makes the following recommendations to lower the risks of cancer and other chronic diseases:

- Eat plenty of vegetables and fruits (at least five servings a day, not including potatoes)
- Replace saturated and trans fats with unsaturated fats (know what you're cooking with; read labels; order healthful foods in restaurants)
- Substitute whole-grain carbohydrates (such as whole-wheat breads and brown rice) for refined-grain carbohydrates (such as white breads and white rice)
- For protein, eat less red meat and processed meats and more nuts, beans, chicken, and fish
- Maintain a stable, healthy weight
- Use alcohol in moderation (it may be beneficial for heart disease but it is not for cancer)
- Exercise regularly and make your day more active

◆ Take one multivitamin daily for insurance (this is most important for those lacking a balanced diet)

Several years after the publication of this book, the FDA issued new dietary guidelines that are in basic agreement with these recommendations (the FDA guidelines can be found at www.mypyramid.gov). Both Dr. Willett and the FDA have made new food pyramids to replace the one designed in 1992. The new pyramids emphasize the importance of exercise and have diminished the recommended intake for carbohydrates in an effort to promote the attainment of an ideal body weight. As of 2009, the old food pyramid, which has carbohydrates at its base (to represent the foundation upon which the other food groups are supported), still remains on bread wrappers and other carbohydrate-based food labels, even though it is clearly outdated.

NUTRITION DURING CANCER TREATMENT

The healthy eating and living guidelines described above are intended for anyone. But people undergoing cancer treatments have special nutritional needs and challenges. Patients who have lost weight from the effects on the body of an untreated cancer will usually regain the weight if effective cancer-fighting therapies are initiated. Appetite stimulants can also be prescribed to promote needed weight gain. I encourage patients who have low body weight caused by other medical problems as well as those expected to lose weight because of side effects from strong cancer treatments to meet with a licensed dietician familiar with the nutritional needs of cancer patients.

If you have cancer, your medical or radiation oncologist will be able to predict the nutritional problems associated with various treatments. The goal should be to develop a nutritional plan to maintain optimal weight during cancer therapy. Intensive dietary counseling has been shown to be the best way to maintain one's nutritional status, enhance one's quality of life, and minimize side effects during strong cancer treatments.

In keeping with our focus on understanding the origins of cancer, I next discuss reasons behind the healthy eating guidelines and why they are thought to help guard against cancer. It is important to note that although diet plays a prominent role in the *prevention* of cancer and in helping patients better tolerate cancer therapies, diet alone has not been shown to be effective as a cancer treatment (see appendix 2 for additional resources).

DIET AND ANTIOXIDANTS

Fruits and vegetables are thought to protect against cancer in large part because of their potent "antioxidant" properties. This term has become synonymous with good health in our culture and is a major way of marketing such foods as ketchup, tea, and juice, to name a few. But what is an antioxidant? Does it counteract an oxidant? Why is it beneficial?

As I discussed earlier, our DNA is continually exposed to damage both from the outside world and from chemicals generated inside a cell during its normal, day-to-day operations. One group of damaging agents is modified forms of oxygen (called "free radicals") that react with healthy proteins, lipids, and DNA to cause oxidative damage or oxidation. When DNA suffers oxidation, its perfect chemical bonds are disrupted and forced to accept an oxygen molecule. This wreaks havoc with the structure of DNA; the result is a DNA mutation. If these mutations occur in tumor suppressor genes or genes that become converted into oncogenes, a cancer can result. Oxidative damage is also involved in inflammation, aging, and vascular disease.

Foods with antioxidant properties help our cells convert the damaging forms of oxygen into innocuous forms, thereby preventing damage to important molecules. Fruits and vegetables have many antioxidant compounds; some of the most commonly discussed compounds are vitamin E, beta-carotene, vitamin C, selenium, and lycopene. Some antioxidant compounds in fruits and vegetables are called carotenoids; these are responsible for the vibrant colors of these plant foods. Lycopene, for example, is the carotenoid in tomatoes that makes them red.

Yet fruits and vegetables contain a host of carotenoids (an orange has more than fifty) that may need to work together to exert their full anti-cancer effect. This may be why studies of people taking individual anti-oxidant supplements, such as vitamin E and beta-carotene, have failed to demonstrate a reduction in cancer; surprisingly, some of these vitamins actually increased the risk of cancer in a number of studies! The most recent disappointment was the large SELECT Study, which failed to demonstrate a benefit for vitamin E or selenium in the prevention of prostate cancer.

Although the potential of natural food supplements to prevent cancer appears vast, much more research is needed to show that taking one or more supplements can be effectively used for this purpose. This point was emphasized in a recent study showing that those with a history of precancerous colon polyps (adenomas removed at routine colonoscopy) who subsequently took 1 milligram a day of folic acid experienced an *increased,* rather than decreased, future risk of developing colon cancer; colon cancer survivors should therefore avoid taking extra folic acid supplements. Overall, experts recommend that antioxidants and essential nutrients be obtained in their natural state by eating the right foods.

One notable exception is vitamin D, adequate levels of which have been associated with a lower risk of developing breast, prostate, colon, and possibly lung cancer. Vitamin D is not an antioxidant; its anticancer effects revolve around its ability to promote the normal growth and maturation of cells. It is essential for preventing osteoporosis in post-menopausal women. Experts recommend that adults take a daily vitamin supplement containing between 800 and 1,000 IU of vitamin D in the form of D3 (cholecalciferol).

OVERWEIGHT AND OBESITY RAISES
THE RISKS FOR CANCER

Excess body fat promotes the development of cancer because it leads to two important changes in the body's chemistry: (1) the development of the so-called insulin resistance syndrome or metabolic syndrome; and (2) the increased production of estrogen.

Insulin resistance and cancer. Fat cells normally release fatty acids into the bloodstream. These molecules can be used for energy and actually compete with glucose as a source of energy by the body. In addition, fatty acids cause chemical changes inside our cells. One important change is making insulin work harder to do its job, that of having glucose transported from the outside to the inside of cells. This situation is termed "insulin resistance," and it often leads to adult-onset diabetes. Insulin resistance forces the body to pump out more insulin in order for cells to receive the glucose they need. As a result, higher levels of insulin are found in the bloodstream, and this in turn causes an increase in related chemicals called insulin-like growth factors (IGFs). High levels of insulin and IGFs create an unhealthy atmosphere for the cells they bathe, promoting heart disease, cancer, obesity, and a shortened life span.

Insulin-like growth factors promote cancer because they enhance the survival and growth of cells and prevent their death. This would be especially unwanted if a cell were to sustain a genetic mutation. Normally, such a cell would be sensed as damaged and targeted for elimination by the body. But in the presence of insulin resistance and high IGF levels, the cell may survive; the damaged cell can then go on to sustain additional DNA mutations that ultimately lead to cancer. In this way excess body weight, through the creation of insulin resistance, promotes the development of cancer.

More fat, more estrogen, more breast cancer. The ovaries are the main source of estrogen production in menstruating women. When ovarian function ceases upon menopause, estrogen is still produced in the female body, although in lesser amounts. In postmenopausal women, fat becomes the main estrogen factory, with higher body weights correlating with higher estrogen levels.

As every woman knows from the experience of menstruation, estrogen stimulates the growth of the breast and uterus. Just as the normal cells in these tissues multiply in response to estrogen, so do (most) cancers derived from them. Therefore, the higher the blood levels of estrogen and related sex hormones, the greater the risk of developing breast and uterine cancer.

Recent studies into how weight affects breast cancer control have shown that women who are overweight at the time of a breast cancer diagnosis and those who gain and retain extra weight after the diagnosis have an increased risk of breast cancer recurrence. The more weight gained, the greater the chances that the cancer may return. It is therefore recommended that women strive hard to maintain weight during breast cancer treatment or lose any weight gained after treatments end.

The connection between fat and breast cancer is in part caused by the fact that fat contains an enzyme called aromatase that increases estrogen production. So even after menopause, when the ovaries have ceased producing estrogen, the hormone still gets made in the body. A class of medicines called aromatase inhibitors (AIs) blocks aromatase from working and thereby drastically reduces the levels of estrogen in the bloodstream. AIs such as femara (Letrozole), anastrazole (Arimidex), and aromasin (Exemestane) are very effective in fighting breast cancer in postmenopausal women, as discussed in chapter 7.

EXERCISE AND CANCER

Regular exercise is a critical part of a healthy pattern for living. Exercise and being physically fit yield tremendous physical, emotional, and mental dividends. Exercise is recommended for cancer patients at all stages of treatment, especially those who have completed cancer therapy. It can maintain strength, improve fatigue, relieve stress, and prevent weight gain, among other benefits. Studies of breast and colon cancer survivors indicate that regular exercise can help prevent a cancer recurrence. The American Cancer Society recommends aerobic exercise (for example, walking, swimming, cycling, taking an exercise class) for at least thirty minutes five days per week.

Cancer treatments may limit a person's ability to exercise. If you are a cancer patient undergoing treatment, you should do less than you think you are capable of and discuss the best time to exercise in relation to your treatments with your oncologist. There will be times when you must rest because of the effects of the cancer or the treatments, when exercise is too difficult to engage in. During these times, short walks, stretching, or gentle yoga may be extremely helpful and not too taxing. Many patients also find that Reiki (a Japanese technique to promote relaxation and healing) and massage can relieve stress and improve movement. Many cancer centers offer these programs, often free of charge or for a nominal fee.

TOBACCO: THE PERFECT CARCINOGEN

In contrast to the difficulties in linking specific foods to the development or prevention of cancer, no such problems exist regarding tobacco. Tobacco products have been proven beyond doubt to induce the changes in normal cells required to convert them into cancerous ones. This has been shown in the laboratory on cells treated with chemicals present in tobacco, in lab animals raised on air filled with tobacco smoke, and in studies of humans who smoke or use any tobacco product—cigarettes, cigars, pipes, chewing tobacco, or snuff. These products are poison because they are full of carcinogens; not even tobacco companies dispute this reality.

It is well established that 90 percent of lung cancers are caused by smoking and that lung cancer is the leading cause of cancer-related death in the United States and worldwide. Yet tobacco also plays a role in bringing about many other cancers: bladder, cervix, esophagus, kidney, larynx, oral/nasal cavity, pancreatic, stomach, and leukemia. It has been estimated that if tobacco were banned, one-third of all cancers in industrialized nations would be eliminated. Talk about a miracle cure!

Why is tobacco such a potent cancer-causing substance? Because it is the perfect carcinogen: it contains chemicals (such as nicotine and NNK, a nitrosamine) that: (1) directly cause mutations in DNA; (2) prevent the damaged cells from dying; and (3) create addiction, causing the user to perpetuate the damage to the body. If these events happen repeatedly, year after year, then the risks that a cancer will form are very high.

But all is not lost, because smokers can benefit from quitting at any time during their lives. For those who smoke but have never had cancer, quitting even at age sixty can add years to their life. For those smokers who have survived cancer, then quitting smoking is one of the best things they can do to prevent another cancer. Moreover, even if smokers are currently battling cancer, then quitting is still very important. Not only will quitting improve their health and their body's ability to tolerate the recommended treatments but they will be improving their chances of survival.

> *Studies suggest that patients with lung cancer who quit smoking live longer than those who continue to smoke.*

Although few studies have been done in other smoking-related cancers, I suspect that they would yield the same results.

Please speak to your doctor in order to get the help you need to quit smoking. If you are a smoker, totally commit yourself to quitting. It is of the utmost importance. Advice on quitting can be found in many places, including doctor's offices, the Internet (such as at www.surgeon-general .gov), and in books.

Why Do Only Some People Get Cancer?

In this chapter thus far, I have described the influence of genetic and environmental factors on the development of cancer. Each has been called a "risk factor" because the specific agent (a gene, a foodstuff) either increases or decreases the risk that cancer will occur. But a risk factor is not a guarantee; it is merely something that raises or diminishes the odds that a cancer will develop. For example, mutations in the BRCA1 gene dramatically raise the risk of breast and ovarian cancer, yet not all who harbor the mutant gene will develop cancer. Although smokers have a twenty times' greater chance of developing lung cancer than nonsmokers, not all smokers will get lung cancer. And lots of people are overweight or obese, get little exercise, and have cancer-prone diets, yet many of them will never get cancer. We must then ask: Why are certain individuals susceptible to a particular cancer risk factor, whereas others are impervious to it? Why do only some people get cancer?

The answer may very well lie within our genes. Although humans are nearly identical at the level of DNA (nearly 99 percent the same), there are of course differences that make each of us unique. One type of difference, called a SNP (single nucleotide polymorphism, pronounced "snip"), represents a single base change to the DNA code that may cause a gene to function slightly differently between individuals. In one person the gene will function at normal levels, whereas in someone with the variation, it may be over- or underactive in its duties in the cell.

Cancer researchers are studying which gene SNPs influence the development of cancer. They are focusing on those that help the body rid itself of environmental toxins, process vitamins such as folic acid (essential for healthy DNA), or repair damaged DNA (gatekeeper and caretaker genes). For example, SNPs in genes called glutathione S-transferases, which detoxify the carcinogens contained in tobacco smoke, may determine why some smokers get lung cancer and others do not: some variants of these genes are better than others at neutralizing the poisons in tobacco. Furthermore, recent discoveries link a tendency to both nicotine addiction and lung cancer with minor variations in the DNA code for the body's nicotine receptors (the cellular targets of nicotine). Thus, as reported in the journal *Nature,* "variants in the sequence of our genome influence not only how we respond to our environment but also our tendency to seek or avoid environment."

Nearly every environmental influence linked to cancer has an effect on our bodies that may be modulated by a number of genes, each with one or more SNP. The number of connections that can be formed is infinite, but only some will be significant. The National Institutes of Health has established the Environmental Genome Project to catalogue how Americans vary genetically in their responses to hazardous environmental chemicals. It is anticipated that, in the not-too-distant future, an individual's "SNP profile" will be available as it relates to cancer susceptibility. Such a profile may tell some people that cooking red meat is extremely harmful to them, others that they need to take high doses of specific vitamins to avoid cancer, and still others that they should eat a lot of cruciferous vegetables to buttress a weak detoxification gene.

In order to achieve this level of individual health care, the most ambitious study of how diet interacts with DNA is under way in Europe, and it is called EPIC, for European Prospective Investigation into Cancer and Nutrition. This study is tracking more than five hundred thousand people in ten European countries, recording their diets in detail and determining the relations between cancer and dietary chemicals, levels of nutrients in the bloodstream, and genetic variation (including SNPs) in nutrition-related genes. With more than nine million samples already collected, this is the largest study of its kind and is yielding an abundance of solid, vital information leading to sound nutritional advice. The findings from the EPIC studies can be followed at http://epic.iarc.fr.

Ultimately, diets, supplements, and medicines will be tailored to each person's unique genetic profile. We are heading to an age of individualized cancer prevention and individualized cancer treatments.

In summary, cancer arises from a complex interplay between our genes and the environment in which we live. Cancer is ultimately a genetic disease, driven by mutations in genes that control the growth, survival, and spread of cells in the body. These mutations are brought on largely by environmental factors, among them diet, lifestyle, and tobacco use. On the flip side, our individual genetic makeup determines how susceptible each of us is to these environmental influences. Still, there will always be cancers that cannot be explained, caused by random errors to DNA and resulting in unspeakable tragedies (such as a twenty-eight-year-old with pancreatic cancer). On a brighter note, the future will bring many new insights into the complicated interactions between our DNA and the world we live in, ultimately leading to a far more satisfying answer to the question "Why did I get cancer?"

Part II

Attacking Cancer

5

How Cancer Grows: The Basis of Cancer Treatments

- A fifty-five-year-old man feels a twinge in his back while golfing. The pain persists and begins to pierce his abdomen. Soon after, he is diagnosed with pancreatic cancer and learns that the tumor is too large to be surgically removed. He asks, "How could I be so sick and not know it? Does cancer grow overnight?"
- A forty-year-old woman with breast cancer undergoes surgery to remove the cancer. Afterward, the surgeon tells her, "The surgery went very well, I got all of it. But you should see the oncologist for chemotherapy." The patient asks, "Why do I need chemo if I'm cancer-free?"
- For four years, a sixty-eight-year-old man with prostate cancer has been receiving hormone treatments that have kept both his cancer and his PSA level (a blood marker of cancer growth) at undetectable levels. Suddenly, the PSA rises and a bone scan shows that the cancer is growing in his bones. He asks, "Why did the medicine stop working? How could the cancer move from my prostate to my bones?"
- A thirty-eight-year-old woman with lymphoma experiences a complete remission of her cancer after two cycles of chemotherapy. She

asks, "Why do I need six cycles of chemo if the cancer is already gone?"

♦ A forty-three-year-old woman with metastatic thyroid cancer involving her lungs is referred to another cancer center for a promising experimental treatment. She returns after a year and informs me that she never received any other treatments despite multiple consultations. I immediately order CT scans, which show that the cancer is no longer present. She asks me, "How can my cancer just disappear?" I reply that it rarely happens and ask if she did anything special to achieve this remarkable result. "Prayed a lot and drank a lot of Gatorade," she said laughingly. "God and Gatorade, who am I to question that?" I replied.

Cancer seems to grow in mysterious ways. It can begin in one location and remain there, or it can spread to other parts of the body. It may grow aggressively from the outset or begin as a slow growth but over time change its stripes and increase rapidly in size. Some cancers remain the same size for long periods, and some can even shrink spontaneously (this is rare except in lymphomas and kidney cancer).

After a successful treatment, cancer may never return and be cured. Alternatively, it may return in the original areas of involvement or in entirely new locations. Again, no two cancer cases behave exactly the same way, and no oncologist has seen every manifestation of every cancer. There are well-described patterns of growth for each cancer type, which is what oncologists are expert at recognizing. But there is a great deal that we do not know about why cancer grows the way it does.

For any individual patient with cancer, it is not possible to predict if and when and in which areas the cancer will grow in the body. Yet just as yesterday's mysteries are common knowledge today, so will today's questions about cancer yield to the light of ongoing scientific sleuthing. Through advances in cancer research, many of the mysteries of cancer growth are becoming more clearly understood. Paralleling these discoveries are improved ways of treating the disease. How cancer grows and how it is treated are closely intertwined. In this chapter I explain how cancer grows in the human body and how this knowledge is shaping the development of modern-day cancer therapies.

Cancer Develops over Decades

One of the first questions that every person turned into a cancer patient asks is, "When did the cancer start?" Anyone diagnosed with cancer naturally wants to know when the disease began, in part to determine if it was caught at its earliest stages but also to try to capture what in their life may have triggered such a revolt in their body.

Most people think of cancer as springing up overnight: one day their body is healthy and the next day there is cancer. They realize that it takes time for the disease to grow to the point of detection, but most think that it begins as a sudden process, an abrupt shock to their healthy cells and tissues. In fact, it is not. Cancers that affect adults usually develop gradually, in stages, and over many years (childhood cancers take less time to develop for a variety of reasons).

The condition that ultimately gets diagnosed as cancer is actually the result of a *series of changes* to one or a few cells that occurred unnoticed over a decade or more. As discussed in chapter 4, this incubation period is shorter for those with a personal, family, and/or genetic predisposition to certain cancers, in whom the disease occurs earlier in life. The development of cancer is often a lengthy and drawn-out process that can be divided into two phases: the precancerous phase and the cancerous phase.

During the precancerous phase of its development, the framework for a cancer is laid in the body. Subtle changes occur to a cell that mark it as different from the surrounding normal cells, such as a new shape or loosened attachments to its neighbors. The affected cell will also begin to multiply. Ultimately, the normal anatomy of the region gives way, and a growth will form, such as a polyp in the lining of the colon or an unusual mole on the surface of the skin. These growths are benign (not cancer), but some types are considered to be precancerous — given enough time, a cancer could develop out of them.

One of the earliest descriptions of precancerous changes was made more than forty years ago, when researchers established a link between smoking and lung cancer. Scientists performed a detailed pathologic study of the lungs of both smokers (some of whom died of lung cancer) and nonsmokers that were available through autopsy at several Veterans Health Administration hospitals in the New York area. They found that the lungs of all smokers, in contrast to those of nonsmokers, were pockmarked with abnormal collections of cells, ranging from the simple to the bizarre (the more bizarre the collection, the likelier it is to become a cancer).

Most important, the more a person smoked, the greater the number of abnormal cells found and the higher the likelihood that lung cancer developed. In fact, the lungs of some smokers, including those who did not die from lung cancer, contained carcinoma in-situ (see chapter 3); presumably, these individuals would soon have developed lung cancer had they not died of other causes. Today researchers are enrolling active and former smokers in clinical trials testing the use of CT scans and PET scans to detect early lung cancer. The hope is that the disease can be caught before it has spread; final recommendations on screening cannot yet be made. It bears repeating that quitting smoking is the best form of cancer prevention.

A similar progression from precancerous changes to full-blown malignancy has been described for nearly every type of cancer. Precancerous abnormalities and early stage cancers of the mouth and throat, breast, colon, skin, prostate, and cervix can be detected effectively with recommended screening tests, whereas others, such as those of the pancreas and ovary, cannot be detected before cancer develops (promising tests are under development).

I must caution against cancer paranoia and overscreening as a means of early detection. Techniques such as full-body CT scanning to detect any abnormal growth in the body or surgical procedures such as the removal of every unusual mole on the skin have not been validated as useful methods of screening for cancer. If a screening test or procedure has not been shown to save lives, and especially if it involves invasive procedures, then its use should be limited to clinical trials that test its true value.

If the precancerous phase goes undetected, some benign growths will morph into a cancer, and the second phase will take hold. The cancerous phase has been estimated as taking eight years for the average breast cancer, which represents the time required for the first bona fide cancer cell to generate a tumor large enough to be detected (one centimeter, roughly a third of an inch, equal to a billion cells). Although every cancer grows at a different speed, this number gives a rough guide as to the duration of the cancerous phase.

If you are a cancer patient, your awareness of the disease begins with the diagnosis and determination of stage; it continues through the estimation of prognosis and the chances for cure, and it culminates with treatment and being a survivor. Yet all of these aspects of cancer revolve around a disease that has been developing in your body for some time.

When a cancer is diagnosed, it represents a particular point in the time line of an abnormal growth, not the beginning of that growth.

It follows then, that when a patient asks me when his or her cancer began, I explain that it likely developed over many years (possibly decades) and in the two phases just described.

Cancer Grows by Organized Chaos

Sharon had little use for doctors. She was in her seventies and had always been healthy. Most members of her family lived into their nineties, and she expected to do the same. She saw her family doctor only for problems and declined recommended cancer-screening tests.

For several weeks Sharon experienced stomach bloating and diarrhea. She began to feel weak and was losing weight. Sensing that something was wrong, she saw her doctor, who performed a fecal blood test, which, if positive, could indicate the presence of colon cancer. The test showed blood in her stool. Sharon was referred to a gastroenterologist for a colonoscopy. Midway through the test, the snakelike "scope" could no longer be advanced because a tumor was blocking it. The biopsy showed cancer; the tumor would have to be removed.

The surgeon removed part of Sharon's colon, including the tumor and many nearby lymph nodes, receptacles for cells draining from the cancer. The pathologist noted that the tumor was an invasive colon cancer (adenocarcinoma) that had spread to several lymph nodes. The main tumor also contained remnants of a benign polyp, called an adenoma. This meant that the invasive cancer developed out of the benign polyp (it also indicated that cancer might have been averted had she undergone a screening colonoscopy). In the final analysis, Sharon had stage III colon cancer, and chemotherapy was recommended in an attempt to prevent her cancer from returning and being a greater threat to her life.

If we could have magically implanted a camera into Sharon's colon twenty years earlier and followed the development of her cancer, what would we have seen? We would have witnessed the gradual advance of a small, benign growth into a large cancer through an organized process called "the polyp cancer sequence" (fig. 11). The polyp cancer sequence is akin to a great tree rising from a small sprout. (A small percentage of colon cancers do not form polyps first but instead form flatter growths, called "flat adenomas," which gastroenterologists can detect during colonoscopy.)

With that magical camera, we would have seen a cell that normally lines the colon wall becoming activated to duplicate itself many times over and grow into a small heap the shape of a broccoli stalk: the polyp. In the beginning, a polyp is small, about the size of a pea. At this early stage, it rarely contains cancer. As the polyp grows, the chances increase that it will harbor cancer, as indicated below:

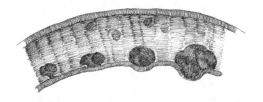

Fig. 11. *Cancer grows in stages*
The inside of the colon, showing how a cancer develops over time from a small to a large polyp, as part of "the polyp cancer sequence." Illustration © Gale V. Parsons.

The Risk of Cancer in a Colon Polyp

Polyp size	Similar to	Chance of harboring cancer
less than 1 cm	pea	less than 1 percent
1–2 cm	grape	5 percent
more than 2 cm	peach pit or bigger	10–20 percent

If large polyps are not removed, a substantial number will pass from the first to the second phase of cancer growth and develop into a malignancy. Once cancer is established inside a polyp, it can grow in two ways: (1) it can expand inside the colon to form a large tumor that interferes with bowel movements and causes symptoms, such as those Sharon experienced; and (2) it can spread to other areas of the body (metastasize), first to nearby lymph nodes and then to such distant organs as the liver.

If we are to find a cure for cancer, then we need specific answers to the following questions:

- What causes the first cell to initiate the polyp sequence?
- What moves it along to enlarge the polyp at each step?
- What ultimately transitions the polyp into cancer?
- What makes the fully formed cancer spread and become a threat to life?

These questions are more commonly phrased in regard to any cancer:

♦ Why did the cancer start?
♦ What makes it grow?
♦ Why do some cancers metastasize?

The answer to all these questions revolves around DNA, which I discussed in chapter 4. The inception, growth, and spread of cancer are interconnected by a common thread, their shared ancestry, their shared DNA.

Cancer Can Grow Unpredictably

Although cancer appears to develop in an organized fashion when viewed from the outside, if we were to go inside a tumor with a little magnifying glass and monitor the movement of cells and the integrity of DNA, we would see a much more chaotic situation. When the first cancer cell duplicates itself to make two cells, it also duplicates its DNA, which gets passed on to its offspring. As two cells become four and so on to generate the billionth cancer cell, the same DNA is duplicated over and over again (remember, a one-centimeter growth contains a billion cells). BUT (this is an important but!), DNA does not remain exactly the same over the lifetime of a cancer.

As a cancer develops and grows, the DNA that guides it along is prone to change. Although the billionth cell is quite similar to the first cell (and would look the same to the pathologist under the microscope), its DNA may have more mutations than the first cell; because DNA determines the functions of every cell, the billionth cell may have different physical properties than the first cell. Thus, as a cancer grows, its genetic makeup becomes diversified, which leads to a diversity of cell types within it. I imagine most readers will be surprised to learn that cancer is not a collection of identical cells.

> *The most critical yet under-discussed property of cancer is its propensity to change and generate cells with different properties.*

The tendency of a cancer to generate cells with different capabilities explains many of the dreadful aspects of cancer that patients find so hard to grapple with: why it can spread from one location to another, why it stops responding to a treatment that was working, and why it can return when it was in remission. The reason is that every cancer, whether it arises in the lung, breast, prostate, bone marrow, fat, or elsewhere, contains different populations of cells that have distinct properties.

Stated another way, the growth of a cancer from one mutant cell is not like putting the original cell on a photocopier, setting the copy number to one billion, and walking away. A cancerous tumor, in fact, does not contain billions of identical clones. Cancer could never develop in this way because it must avoid the immune system's attack on it, live in areas of low oxygen tension, and compete with the rest of the body for vital nutrients. As these conditions change in the body, a cancer must adapt; if it fails to adapt, it is eliminated.

Inside any tumor are cells that are living and cells that have died. There are cancer cells capable of reproducing many others, called cancer stem cells, and cells completely devoid of this capacity. Cancer's diversity is generated early. By the time it is diagnosed, some cells *may* already be capable of metastasizing and others may be able to withstand a particular cancer treatment. This is the basis of cancer's resistance to treatment.

Cancer Is Survival of the Fittest

Nature dictates that in any environment, survival is awarded to those best suited to it. The physical and mental capabilities of any species are determined largely by their DNA. Cancer can also be thought of as abiding by this principle of "survival of the fittest," a phrase coined based on the work of Charles Darwin. A cancer survives only by generating cells that are fit enough to grow in the face of the body's restrictions (listed above) and the arsenal of cancer-fighting therapies to which we subject it.

Another word for a cancer cell is clone. When new cancer cells or clones are generated inside a tumor, some will be hearty enough to survive and others will not be. The heartiest ones will expand in number until they encounter something that limits their growth, such as a cancer-fighting drug. If some cells survive the treatment, then it is mainly because their DNA contains the necessary alterations that help them resist the drug; this population of cells will then expand, and the composition of the cancer will again change.

Thus, the makeup of a cancer is dynamic, punctuated by periods of growth and periods of dormancy, responsive both to random changes to its DNA and to the changing nature of its environment. This propensity of cancer cells to adapt, just like living species in nature, has been termed "clonal evolution." Clonal evolution enhances a cancer's range of abilities and explains a great deal about its behavior.

For example, when a cancer returns after being declared in complete remission, it is because a few cells were different enough to stay alive after a treatment killed nearly all the other cells; this difference could have been present from the start of treatment or it could have developed as a response to it. Whichever occurred, it is cancer's ability to diversify and adapt its DNA that enables it to survive (fig. 12).

We can now answer the essential questions posed above: it is by virtue of cancer's propensity to change—changing DNA, leading to cells with new abilities—that a polyp goes through its cancer sequence and that any cancer first develops and then behaves the way it does in the body.

The Devil Is in the Details

The types of changes to DNA that enable a cancer to grow, survive, and evolve can be understood by describing the development of colon cancer. The first DNA mutation that starts a cell on the long road to

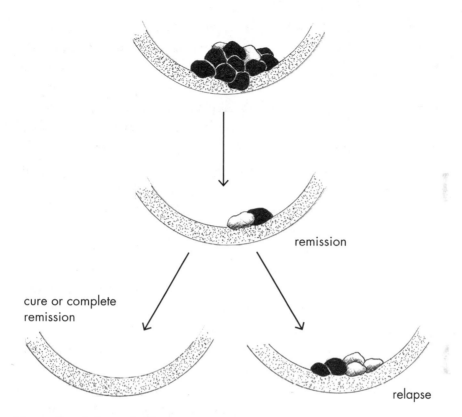

Fig. 12. *Remission and relapse*
A cancer contains a mixture of cells (top), which reduce in number in response to treatment (middle), resulting in remission. If all cells are eradicated, there is complete remission (bottom left), whereas if the cancer grows back, a relapse is experienced (bottom right). Illustration © Gale V. Parsons.

becoming a colon cancer is caused by a combination of environmental factors (such as a diet low in fiber and high in red meat) and a person's genetic makeup. With additional genetic changes, a benign polyp emerges. Further changes cause the polyp to be converted into a cancer. Still more mutations to DNA enable the mature cancer to leave the confines of the colon and spread to lymph nodes, the liver, and other locales. The conquest of cancer begins with the precise understanding of these changes to DNA, a fact not lost on science's brightest minds.

Dr. Bert Vogelstein and colleagues have pioneered our understanding of the genetic changes that bring about cancer. They have clarified that most cancers proceed according to a "genetic model" in which each step on the road to cancer is accompanied by additional DNA alterations. Many of these alterations involve the activation of oncogenes and loss of tumor suppressor genes, which I described in chapter 4 as being central to the development of every cancer.

The multitude of DNA changes that characterize cancer explains why the disease often needs to be treated with more than one drug: many methods of attack are needed to hit so many different targets. For example, a patient with advanced colon cancer today may receive up to four medicines as the initial effort to control the disease: three chemotherapy drugs (5-FU and leucovorin plus either irinotecan or oxaliplatin) plus bevacizumab (Avastin), a targeted therapy that alters blood flow to a tumor. Ongoing clinical trials are testing the addition of still more drugs to the standard four-drug colon cancer regimen. In the future colon cancer treatment may involve the use of five or six drugs in an attempt to eliminate every last cancer cell.

The treatment of other cancers is following suit. The addition of newer targeted drugs to traditional chemotherapy is leading patients to have a better quality of life, longer survivals, and more cures. Also, the addition of radiation therapy to chemotherapy ("chemoradiation") to fight cancers that are difficult to cure surgically, such as stage III cancers of the lung, pancreas, and esophagus, provides a multipronged assault on cancer's many deranged pathways of growth and survival. Sometimes, and in particular with cancer, you have to fight fire with fire.

Cancer's development has both organized and chaotic aspects. As chaos affects its genetic makeup, a cancer generates a diversity of cells with varying abilities. Ultimately, some cells may spread and cause metastases, the greatest challenge to survival. This is the subject of the next chapter.

6

Cancer Treatments Revolve around Metastasis

Anyone who has tried to learn about cancer soon realizes that the disease and the drugs used to combat it are overwhelmingly complicated. Yet the vast world of cancer drug therapy mainly revolves around one aspect: metastasis. Metastasis is the process by which a cancer spreads from its origin to other locations in the body; "metastases" represent the tumors in these distant locales. Cancer treatments center on the principle that metastases need to be either treated or prevented. This is because the presence of cancer in regions beyond its original location often does the most harm.

Many cancers are first treated with surgery or radiation. The goal of these treatments is to achieve what is called "local control": the elimination of the cancer where it arose so that it cannot regrow and cause problems. If it has not already spread elsewhere in the body, then these measures lead to a cure.

In contrast, if detectable metastases are present at diagnosis or if the diagnosis is a blood or lymph system cancer, the priority turns from local control to control of the cancer throughout the body. Surgery will be more limited or avoided entirely.

129

If a patient is undergoing regular cancer drug treatments (which can range from a daily pill to intermittent intravenous chemotherapy), then he or she is working either to eliminate metastases found at diagnosis or to prevent their future development. A third group of patients has to deal with an intermediate situation: a cancer that has grown too extensively for surgical removal but has not yet formed detectable metastases in distant sites. These scenarios outline the three broad categories of cancer drug treatments, which we can categorize by their relation to surgery.

The Three Categories of Cancer Drug Treatments
1. After surgery
   Name: *Adjuvant* therapy
   Goal: Prevent the growth of undetectable metastases into measurable tumors
2. Before surgery
   Name: *Neoadjuvant* therapy
   Goal: Shrink bulky cancers to improve surgical outcomes
3. Instead of surgery
   Name: None
   Goal: Treat metastases present at the time of diagnosis

In the following sections, I explain the rationale for each of the three categories of cancer treatments, addressing the most common concerns that patients have about them. For purposes of clarity, I provide examples of how certain cancers are treated with a particular sequence of chemotherapy, radiation, or surgery. It is important to understand, however, that there may be several acceptable ways to treat a cancer; researchers continuously strive to improve on current methods through clinical trials. No specific recommendations regarding the treatment of any cancer should be drawn from the examples I cite. The optimal treatment of any cancer is determined through discussions with your physicians.

After Surgery: "Why Do I Need Chemo If I'm Cancer-Free?"

No one really wants to meet with an oncologist if they don't have to (I don't take this personally). Patients who undergo cancer surgery of course hope that the surgeon will come to their bedside after the operation and say, "Well, that's it. I got everything, you're cured. Go on with the rest of your life. This cancer won't be bothering you again." In reality, many patients will hear something like this: "The surgery went very well. I got all the cancer. But you should meet with an oncologist in case you need chemotherapy." All told, nearly a third of cancer patients undergo cancer treatment after surgery, called adjuvant therapy, as part of a plan to cure their cancer (*Webster's* defines "adjuvant" as "a person or thing that helps").

Adjuvant therapy may consist of drug and/or radiation treatments. Radiation is given to the region from which a cancer was removed in order to decrease the chances that the cancer will return there (prevent a local relapse); examples include breast radiation after lumpectomy, lung radiation after removal of a lung tumor, and brain radiation after resection of a brain tumor. In contrast, drug therapies attack cancer cells wherever they may be in the body in an effort to prevent isolated pockets of cells from developing into detectable metastases (this process is called "distant relapse").

Many patients wonder why they should subject themselves to the side effects of drugs and radiation if the surgeon told them that the cancer was completely removed. The reason is that having a primary cancer removed is not always the same as being rendered "cancer-free." The surgeon removed only the cancer that he or she could see. In many cancers, however, small clusters of cells escape into the blood or lymphatic system before the cancer is diagnosed and removed. These microscopic deposits of cancer, called "occult metastases" or "micrometastases," cannot be detected reliably by current methods and can eventually grow to form detectable or visible tumors in the liver, lungs, bones, and other regions of the body.

> *The goal of adjuvant therapy is to destroy micrometastases so that they can never develop into tumors.*

Adjuvant therapy is often successful because it is easier to eradicate micrometastases than it is to eliminate overt metastases. In other words, the same type of cancer treated with the same drugs can be cured more often when metastases are microscopic than when they have become obvious and measurable. The reasons for this are not known with certainty but have to do with how much more efficiently cancer therapies penetrate small tumors and the greater likelihood of drug resistance as a cancer enlarges, owing to clonal evolution (discussed in chapter 5).

For example, when chemotherapy is used to treat patients with stage IV lung cancer, it leads to a modest improvement in survival, and cures occur only in a small percentage of cases. But when the same chemotherapy (vinorelbine and cisplatin) was recently used in a study of patients with early-stage lung cancer, who are at risk to develop metastases, 69 percent of the patients treated with chemotherapy were alive at five years, compared to 54 percent of patients who received no chemotherapy after surgical removal of the cancer. Overall, chemotherapy decreased the risk of death by more than 30 percent. What this information means is that for a number of patients in whom lung cancer was destined to return and take their lives, chemotherapy (and radiation in some cases) made all the difference and stopped this process in its tracks. I encourage all patients to meet with a medical oncologist after undergoing surgical removal of lung cancer in order to discuss the benefits and risks of adjuvant therapy.

An equally dramatic advance was reported in 2005 for the adjuvant treatment of breast cancer. Approximately 20 percent of breast cancers produce a protein, called Her2, in high amounts, which stimulates the cancer to grow. A targeted drug therapy called trastuzumab (Herceptin), which attaches to Her2 and blocks it from working, has been used since 1998 to treat stage IV (metastatic) breast cancer. In this setting and especially when combined with chemotherapy, Herceptin prolongs life and often reduces the amount of cancer but cannot eradicate it.

Yet when Herceptin and chemotherapy were given as adjuvant therapy for earlier stages of breast cancer, something remarkable occurred. Several large clinical trials performed around the world demonstrated that women with Her2-positive breast cancer who received Herceptin either with or following chemotherapy had a dramatically reduced risk of cancer relapse than those who received chemotherapy alone. It appears that the Herceptin and chemotherapy combination provides a crucial one-two knock-out blow to Her2 breast cancer that neither can provide alone. In short, many individuals in whom breast cancer was destined to return had their destinies powerfully and positively altered: micrometastases were killed so that cancer relapses were averted.

These recent results highlight the fact that cancer therapies are continually improving; recommendations for the adjuvant treatment of cancer change every few years depending on the results of the latest clinical trials. They also demonstrate the vital importance of good clinical trials and the enthusiastic participation of both patients and physicians in this process.

Eye on the Prize: Complete Cancer Eradication

The use of adjuvant therapy is relatively new, having first come into widespread use after a 1975 clinical trial demonstrated that patients with breast cancer who received a chemotherapy pill, called melphalan, had fewer distant cancer relapses than those who received no further treatment after surgery (the standard of care at that time). Before this study, doctors were powerless to prevent metastases from developing after surgery.

In the thirty years since that landmark study, remarkable progress has been made in the adjuvant treatment of many cancers, especially breast cancer. A number of new chemotherapy drugs have been discovered, such as Taxol and Taxotere, and combined with older drugs with greater effectiveness; these treatments are often referred to by their initials, such as "A-C-T," which stands for Adriamycin, Cytoxan, and Taxol; "T-C," for Taxotere and Cytoxan; and "C-M-F," for Cytoxan, Methotrexate, and 5-FU (5-fluorouracil). Many other adjuvant chemotherapy regimens to treat breast cancer are in use and under development.

In addition, breast cancer adjuvant therapy may include hormone therapies such as tamoxifen or an aromatase inhibitor (anastrazole, aromasin, letrozole) that may be recommended either following or instead of chemotherapy. Hundreds of thousands of women have bravely and generously participated in clinical research that has allowed the continued refinement of breast cancer adjuvant therapy. Such research will continue with even greater gusto as new biologic agents like Herceptin are tested in this setting.

> *Whether a patient receives chemotherapy, hormone therapy, a targeted agent, or combinations of these medicines after surgery, the goal remains the same: to cure the cancer by preventing the growth of micrometastases.*

It is a powerful notion that in the day-to-day routine of swallowing a little pill such as tamoxifen or an aromatase inhibitor, breast cancer patients are helping to kill any cancer cells that may be present in their bodies and prevent a cancer relapse.

There has also been considerable progress in the adjuvant therapy of cancers other than those affecting the breast and lung. Treatment of stage III colon cancer (involving nearby lymph nodes) with chemotherapy after surgery has raised the five-year survival rate from 55 percent to nearly 80 percent, and new agents will likely push cure rates even higher. Adjuvant hormone therapy of high-risk prostate cancer after treatment with surgery or radiation leads to fewer cancer relapses and longer survivals. Either chemotherapy or radiation or both are commonly used after surgery for many cancers.

I wish to make two final important points about adjuvant therapy. First, the timing and dosages of the drugs should be maintained at their recommended schedules. Although cancer treatments can sometimes be adjusted to diminish their side effects, this practice should be avoided during adjuvant therapy because the goal is cure. Certainly, if severe side effects occur, the treatment regimen will be modified; the oncologist will make the necessary changes. Products that support the blood system during chemotherapy, such as Neupogen and Neulasta, may be necessary to ensure that full doses of chemotherapy are administered.

Second, it is impossible to determine the effectiveness of adjuvant treatment for any individual. It is natural for a patient to ask after cancer therapy, "How do I know if it worked?" In the case of adjuvant therapy, there are no tumors to measure. The simplest way to think of this is that if the cancer never returns, then the treatment accomplished its task (or metastases were never destined to develop). If the cancer does relapse, the treatment was not effective enough.

When Surgery Is Not the First Step

In many cases of cancer, surgery is not the best initial treatment. And sometimes surgery is best avoided altogether. Although most patients diagnosed with cancer naturally "want the cancer out," this may not always be possible or in their best interests. The three main situations when this is the case are:

1. The cancer is in a critical location, and removing it would lead to an important loss of function
2. The cancer is too extensive to be removed easily
3. The cancer has already metastasized

Each situation is discussed below.

THE CANCER IS IN A CRITICAL LOCATION

A cancer can sometimes grow in such a vital part of the body that an operation to remove it would result in permanent disability, disfigurement, or even death. For example, surgical treatment of advanced can-

cers of the larynx (voice box) requires removal of the larynx (laryngec-
tomy), which results in loss of the ability to speak. Surgical removal of a
bone tumor may require amputation, resulting in loss of a limb; resection of a cancer of the rectum may require the rerouting of feces to an
external bag (colostomy).

In all of these situations and others, oncologists have developed
"organ preservation" treatments that seek to avoid surgery in order to
treat the cancer. These treatments usually involve both chemotherapy
and radiation, often given at the same time. If organ preservation fails
to eradicate the cancer, surgery can then be performed in an attempt to
do so. The recommendation to administer chemotherapy and radiation
rather than surgery as the primary way to treat a cancer is arrived at
jointly by the medical, surgical, and radiation oncologists involved in a
case.

THE CANCER IS TOO LOCALLY
ADVANCED TO BE REMOVED EASILY

Sometimes a cancer is large by the time it is diagnosed; at other times the
primary cancer may not be big but nearby lymph nodes containing cancer are large. Both situations refer to cancers that are "locally advanced,"
meaning that they have not formed detectable distant metastases but
have grown rather extensively in the region where they arose. Such cancers usually fall within stage III (stages I and II are localized, whereas
stage IV is disseminated cancer; see chapter 2). In these situations, were
surgery to be performed first, it would have to be either very extensive,
removing large areas of normal tissue, or less than complete in entirely
removing the cancer.

Increasingly, surgeons and medical oncologists are first recommend-
ing chemotherapy (and often radiation) in order to shrink locally advanced cancers and make them easier to remove. A cancer treatment
that is given before surgery is called neoadjuvant or induction therapy.

The modern-day treatment of rectal cancer is an excellent example of
how neoadjuvant therapy can greatly diminish the extent of surgery re-

quired. In the past, many patients with rectal cancer first underwent extensive surgery, which required a permanent colostomy. Today, patients with large rectal tumors (T3 or T4) or lymph node involvement (detected by rectal ultrasound) will typically first be prescribed a course of radiation to the pelvis given along with chemotherapy in order to shrink the cancer. A good result enables the surgeon to remove a limited area of the rectum, leaving the patient with intact bowel and no colostomy. But the treatment is still not done! Adjuvant chemotherapy will then be given after surgery in an attempt to eradicate micrometastases throughout the body and cure the patient.

Other examples of cancers that may be treated with induction chemotherapy include certain locally advanced cancers of the lung, esophagus, prostate, bladder, breast, and head and neck regions. In contrast to cancer treated in the adjuvant setting, locally advanced cancers can often be seen or felt and cause symptoms: a large breast mass may cause pain and psychological distress, a lung cancer may cause shortness of breath and cough, and an esophagus cancer may cause difficulty eating and weight loss. It is very gratifying for the physician and a hopeful sign for the patient to witness a large breast mass shrink, breathing become easier, and the ability to eat restored as the treatments do their job.

Sometimes neoadjuvant treatments work so well that they drive the cancer into a complete remission: pathology analysis of the surgical specimen obtained after treatment reveals no evidence of living cancer cells. This does not guarantee that the cancer is cured and will not return; local recurrences or distant metastases may still arise at a later date. Yet patients who do experience a pathologic complete remission have a greater chance of being cured than those who do not because chemotherapy that wipes out all the cancer cells in a primary tumor may have the same effect on micrometastases throughout the body.

One prominent exception to the neoadjuvant therapy approach to locally advanced cancers is ovarian cancer. Most women with ovarian cancer are diagnosed when the disease has spread to many areas of the abdominal cavity. Despite this, surgery is usually performed first because removal of as much disease as possible (called "optimal debulking") improves both how a patient feels and the response to subsequent chemotherapy. Exceptions exist here, too; some women with ovarian cancer may need chemotherapy before surgery in order to decrease the bulk of the cancer and improve their overall health. To quote my own mantra, "There's nothing simple about cancer!'"

INOPERABLE CANCERS

The role of preoperative therapy is to shrink locally advanced cancers in order to make them more easily removed at surgery. But not all such cancers are amenable to this approach. Some have grown to such a degree that their removal may not be feasible despite the many advances in surgical techniques; an example would be a large brain tumor. Some cancers, therefore, are better off being treated *only* with chemotherapy and radiation. Surgery is best avoided in these situations because it would not lead to cure or the best outcome.

Surgeons and other cancer experts have established specific criteria for each cancer to determine its operability. These criteria focus on determining if cancer has spread to particular lymph node regions or if the cancer encroaches on nearby blood vessels or other organs. This determination often requires additional testing, such as MRI, PET scan, or endoscopy with ultrasound (for gastrointestinal cancers) and biopsies of suspect lymph nodes. Sometimes even a minioperation such as laparoscopy will be performed so that the surgeon can visually inspect the extent of disease before deciding to proceed with a large operation (this is most commonly performed for pancreatic cancer).

If the above tests show that the cancer is limited in its extent and can be surgically removed with a chance for cure, then the surgeon will recommend an operation. If the tests reveal that the cancer has spread too far to be removed for cure, then it is deemed inoperable or "unresectable."

The terms "inoperable" and "unresectable" do not always mean that a surgeon *could* not remove a locally advanced cancer; certainly, in the days before modern chemotherapy and radiation, surgeons tried to cure bulky cancers with heroic surgery (such as the disfiguring operation for breast cancer called the radical mastectomy, which removed chest wall muscles as well as the overlying breast). Rather, these terms mean that other approaches have been shown to be superior to surgery in terms of improving a patient's quality of life and extending survival.

For example, if a pancreatic cancer is growing into nearby major blood vessels or if a lung cancer has spread to lymph nodes on both sides of the mediastinum (stage IIIB), then extensive surgery to clear out all the cancer will not be performed. Instead, in these and similar situations affecting the esophagus, cervix, throat, and others, chemoradiation will be recommended as the "definitive" treatment; the radiation will encompass the entire extent of the cancer while the chemotherapy helps the radiation beams kill cancer cells more effectively.

Still, there are nuances here as well, and surgery may ultimately be helpful in certain initially unresectable cancers. For example, pancreatic cancer that appears to be pressing against local blood vessels rather than extensively wrapping around them may become surgically removable after a course of chemoradiation. As always, the specific details of each case determine the range of treatment options.

New research protocols aim to integrate targeted therapies (see chapter 7) into traditional chemoradiation protocols in order to improve survivals across the spectrum of cancers too advanced to be surgically removed.

THE CANCER HAS METASTASIZED

Metastases can be present when a cancer is diagnosed or manifest at some time after the cancer has been treated, constituting a cancer relapse. Regardless of when they are detected, being informed that one's cancer has metastasized is devastating news, rivaled only by cancer's first declaration. BUT it is essential to take stock of the situation, understand the diagnosis, extent of metastases (many or a few), treatment options, and possible outcomes.

Some stage IV cancers are curable, although most have a low chance of complete eradication and cure. If cure is not a likely outcome, prolonged survival may be attainable through control of the cancer with treatments administered over months or years. If the patient chooses no treatment, most commonly because the outlook is poor and he or she does not feel that the possible benefits of therapy outweigh the risks, then good supportive care (as provided by hospice) should be sought out to maximize the patient's comfort and quality of life.

Yet today many people are living full and active lives while under treatment for metastatic cancer. Treatments may be given intermittently whenever the cancer flares or on a continuous basis. Furthermore, new hope springs yearly as novel weapons to fight cancer are introduced. *As always, remember that every patient and every cancer is unique.*

> *To maximize survival in the case of a metastatic cancer, it is important to consider all the treatment options available and to exercise each option at the right time.*

Metastatic Disease: Cure versus Control

The mainstay of treatment of metastatic cancers is drug therapy. Whether they are injected or swallowed, drugs travel throughout the body to reach cancer cells wherever they are hiding. These treatments may be administered for brief or extended periods, depending on the type of cancer and goal of treatment. Treatment "goals" are defined by what can be realistically achieved given all available and experimental approaches. Although cure is always desired, the reality is that the best we can hope for with many cancers is long-term control.

A patient's oncologist will make the goals of treatment clear. The two examples that follow illustrate the approaches to treating cancer for cure or for control.

THE NATURE LOVER

Robin, a forty-five-year-old woman with an affinity for natural healing and a love of animals, feels a mass in her abdomen one day. After testing, she is ultimately diagnosed with stage IV non-Hodgkin's lymphoma involving the liver. She undergoes six courses (cycles) of chemotherapy plus an immune therapy (CHOP-Rituxan, see chapter 3), followed by small doses of chemotherapy administered by spinal tap into her spinal fluid to prevent lymphoma from growing in her central nervous system. The treatment is hard. She loses her hair and at various times experiences weakness, nausea, pain, and discomfort. But three months later she is back to work, feeling well, with a new short hairdo. Four years later, Robin remains cancer-free and has much longer hair.

THE PAINTER

Patrick, a seventy-year-old accomplished painter, is diagnosed with stage IV prostate cancer involving his bones five years after he underwent surgical removal of the prostate. He is treated by his urologist with injections of a hormone-blocking drug (Lupron) every four months to keep the cancer in check. After two years, the PSA (blood marker of cancer growth) rises again, and he is prescribed a pill (Casodex) to block the ability of testosterone to fuel the cancer. By this time, Patrick has stopped painting, mainly from depression at the thought of dying soon. He is referred to me for management of his cancer at this point.

The new medicine lowers the PSA for six months, but then the PSA begins to rise again, and a bone scan shows worsening of the cancer. The Casodex is stopped, but the PSA continues to rise (it can sometimes fall in this situation). Patrick learns that his estimated average survival at this point is approximately two years. He begins another hormone-blocking pill called ketoconazole; the PSA plummets to the normal range, and he feels well. He begins to paint again and even travels abroad for inspiration. After a year and a half, the PSA begins to rise swiftly, and Patrick feels weak; he stops painting.

We change treatment to intravenous injections of the chemotherapy drug Taxotere, given once every three weeks. The PSA steadily declines and after six treatments is close to the normal range. The chemotherapy tires him for about a week, leaving two good weeks out of every three to accomplish things. After eight cycles, the treatment is put on hold to give him a break from therapy and liberate him from frequent office visits and needle-sticks. Patrick does not feel that he is dying anymore; he travels, paints, and enjoys the company of his loved ones.

After six months, the cancer again becomes active, and he resumes treatment in a clinical trial testing a new drug. The situation remains stable for a few months but then requires that he go back on chemotherapy. The cancer responds, and his condition improves once again. It is now three years since he expected to live between "one and two." Patrick knows the cancer cannot be cured. He knows he will need to be on and off treatment for the rest of his life. But, he says, "I am so grateful. I didn't expect to be here now. I don't know how much time I have but, life on the whole is very good."

TO CURE OR CONTROL?

Robin's cancer story is brief, her treatment well defined. The treatment course could be mapped out for her at the outset. If the cancer responded completely, as we had hoped, then she would not require other therapies. Although the treatment was arduous, toward the end of it, Robin could look forward to its completion and "getting on with my life." Although cure was not a guarantee, it was a distinct possibility. Metastatic or advanced stages of cancers treated with the *strong* possibility of cure (more than 50 percent of the time) include aggressive non-Hodgkin's lymphomas, Hodgkin lymphoma, testicular cancer, and some rare tumors. Advanced stages of ovarian cancer are also treated for cure with chemotherapy after surgery; the five-year survival rate is approximately 35 percent.

Patrick's journey is longer. It is also the road more traveled by people who live with cancer. Control of his cancer required a series of treatments given for unpredictable periods of time and in an unpredictable sequence. The different treatments available could be listed at the outset, but when each option would be used could not be foretold; it would depend on how effective each was. We could not have known that the ketoconazole would work for as long as it did; in some patients it works for a shorter time or not at all and chemotherapy is instituted sooner. As one of my colleagues likes to tell his patients with metastatic disease, the control of their cancer will be "a work in progress."

The key word is *control:* control of cancer that we do not yet know how to cure. This control is achieved through treatments given at the appropriate times over months or, we hope, years. Because good control converts incurable cancers into chronic conditions that must be dealt with for the remainder of one's life, I will refer to them as chronic cancers. In a small percentage of patients (usually less than 3 percent), treatment may lead to complete remission of the cancer and eventual cure of breast, lung, colon, or other cancers. But because the percentage of patients cured of "incurable cancers" is so low, most oncologists refrain from mentioning this possibility out of fear that such information could give their patients false hope and unrealistic expectations. In my practice I do discuss cure as a potential outcome (and always hope for it), although I emphasize its rarity; if the cancer remains undetectable as time marches on, a patient will find that his or her oncologist is more receptive to a discussion of cure.

Despite the above, extensive research has so far failed to find easy cures or even difficult ones for many cancers. Efforts to blast away metastatic cancer with megadoses of chemotherapy have fallen short because they do not root it out but rather cause more harm than good: the cancer is still present and the patient is sicker than ever. Not surprisingly, those cancers that can be cured by such an approach are the ones most responsive to standard doses of chemotherapy, namely the blood and lymph cancers (high-dose chemotherapy followed by return of one's own blood stem cells, to reconstitute blood formation, is an effective treatment for multiple myeloma and relapsed lymphoma, as well as some cases of testicular cancer and pediatric cancers).

> *Ultra-aggressive efforts that have failed to cure metastatic cancers have given way to smarter ways of administering cancer treatments that are both more effective and less toxic.*

These new efforts include: (1) the use of smaller doses of chemotherapy given more frequently; for example, one can give a hundred units of a drug every three weeks or thirty-three units weekly (as long as studies support their equivalence). The lower dose given more often tends to be less harsh on normal tissues, but the tumor "sees" the same total dose intensity over a three-week period; and (2) the development of targeted therapies that, by blocking specific pathways of cancer growth, enhance the effectiveness of chemotherapy.

When Chief Justice William Rehnquist was diagnosed with aggressive thyroid cancer and at the age of eighty returned to work rather than retire, many in Washington and the media were shocked. This prompted *New York Times* editor Janet Battaile to write a piece entitled, "Very Much Alive, Thank You." Battaile disclosed that she was very much alive and a five-year survivor of multiple myeloma currently under treatment with thalidomide. She wrote about a number of prominent legislators and judges who were also working and thriving while receiving treatment for cancer; they called themselves "the chemo kids."

There is no doubt that oncologists like myself the world over are caring for an ever-growing number of inspiring individuals who are living longer and better despite harboring active cancer. Our community cancer center is a bustling celebration of life rather than a somber, sterile environment; the struggle is evident and emotions are raw at times, to be sure, but an atmosphere created by genuine human warmth and caring makes everyone's task lighter.

It is not my intention to paint an overly rosy picture in which all patients with such cancers are now living many years. It is no secret that Judge Rehnquist did eventually die from his cancer. As an oncologist, I have the frankly disturbing but solemn responsibility of caring for too many people who lose their life to this disease.

It is not acceptable that we cure too few advanced cancers. Even though billions of dollars are invested in cancer research every year, most new drugs in the research pipeline will extend life rather than be silver bullets that pierce the heart of cancer. But this is still progress (the money is well spent!), and it is important to keep in mind that, by their very nature, advances in research are incremental. We are always elated, of course, when the murmuring momentum of research is jolted by a breakthrough that dramatically improves the lives of those battling cancer.

Between hope and hype, there is reality in which research gains are hard-won and modest and cancer must be battled with grit. This is the fight of your life.

CONTROL OF CHRONIC CANCERS

Throughout this book, I have made the case that each of us is unique and that every cancer is unique. Every cancer patient is also at a unique point in his or her life when diagnosed, having gotten there by a life journey that no one else could have traveled. Some are in the prime of their life, with dependents and the bitter need to survive, others at a ripe age, with their life goals accomplished and an acceptance of life's limits. All of these factors and the cold, hard facts about the cancer at hand go into formulating a plan of action to treat a chronic cancer. Not surprisingly, this plan differs from patient to patient.

Perhaps this last statement is surprising or unsettling. After all, shouldn't there be a "best" treatment for any disease, especially one as serious as cancer? For the highly curable cancers, usually there are just one or two best treatments; this is the case mainly because once a curative, well-tolerated therapy is found through years of trial and error, it is difficult to improve upon. For example, most patients with testicular cancer requiring chemotherapy will receive one of two regimens, PEB or EP (P = platinum, E = etoposide, B = blemoycin).

On the other hand, the treatment of less curable, chronic cancers includes not one or two best possibilities but an expanding array of equally effective choices (a patient may receive different expert opinions on treatment; none can be considered the "right" treatment). Just ten years ago, the oncologist could reach for only a few chemotherapy drugs. Today there are many new chemotherapy drugs plus better ways of giving older ones; a growing list of targeted therapies; combinations of chemo and targeted treatments; and experimental drugs being tested in clinical trials that have a greater likelihood of being successful than in years past.

For example, as of 2009, a woman with metastatic breast cancer may receive one of seven hormone-blocking drugs (for many years there was mainly tamoxifen or Megace); when one stops working, another one is employed. She may receive one of more than ten chemotherapy drugs or as many combinations of them; again, when one stops working, another option is tapped. In addition, if the cancer expresses the Her2 protein, then the targeted therapies Herceptin or lapatinib (Tykerb) are added to chemotherapy. If the cancer does not make Her2, bevacizumab (Avastin) may be added to chemotherapy (how these drugs work to stop cancer growth is explained in chapter 7). Each new drug and every new combination represent another way to keep the cancer in check. Each advance came about through cancer research: new drugs were discovered and tested in altruistic and brave cancer patients in clinical trials.

The same principles hold true for other cancers, whether they are the common ones such as lymphoma, lung, colon, and prostate cancer or the less common ones such as sarcomas and kidney or pancreatic cancer. Although the treatment well runs dry faster for the less common cancers, even this stagnant ground is shifting as new options are in the offing. As I wrote this section, two new drugs, sorafenib (Nexavar) and sunitinib (Sutent), were approved by the FDA for metastatic kidney cancer and a third, called temsirolimus (Torisel), was approved as this book neared publication. Kidney cancer is largely unresponsive to chemotherapy drugs. Before the introduction of these targeted therapies, treatment options for kidney cancer included mainly interferon and interleukin, which work with minimal success.

Clearly, the treatment landscape for advanced cancers is undergoing a revolution. The ultimate goal of cancer research is to find cures; the immediate goal for cancer patients with metastatic disease is disease control, long-term survival, and an acceptable quality of life. These are being increasingly realized through the use of all available options: effective approved treatments and promising experimental ones. Yet whichever therapy is chosen to treat a chronic cancer, the goal should always be to give the most effective therapy with the fewest side effects whenever possible.

How a Treatment Strategy Is Chosen

Among the available options for the treatment of a cancer, the oncologist will choose one to start with ("first-line therapy"), another as a second-line therapy when needed, and then others as dictated by the behavior of the cancer. These choices will be guided by several factors:

FACTORS ONCOLOGISTS CONSIDER
IN CHOOSING A TREATMENT

The data. Oncologists love data, and the treatment of cancer is guided more by the results of clinical trials than any other field of medicine (this is a good thing, producing orderly and methodical progress). Every year at the main meeting of oncologists run by the American Society of Clinical Oncology, nearly ten thousand new studies are presented from around the world pertaining to the biology, treatment, and prevention of cancer (see appendix 2 for web sites). The American Society of Hematology runs the corresponding meeting for blood disorders. Besides these and many other meetings, the latest cancer research is published in many medical journals. In addition, research leaders in each cancer field meet frequently to discuss the latest findings with other oncologists and to draft guidelines on treating various cancers. Oncologists use a range of data and information when deciding on the best treatment to give a patient. These include: definitive results from large, randomized clinical trials, in which a new treatment is compared to the current standard of care; less certain but "promising" results from smaller studies;

the recommendation of a colleague who may have special expertise in treating a particular cancer; and their own experience.

Important biologic properties of the cancer. In addition to the grade and other features described in a standard pathology report (such as the presence of the estrogen receptor and Her2 in breast cancers), additional studies may be performed that guide treatment decisions. These may include specific molecules or genetic alterations that the cancer possesses. For example, if a lung cancer contains a mutation in the DNA code of the EGFR gene, then the pill erlotinib (Tarceva) may be highly effective and used instead of chemotherapy. Or if a colon or rectal cancer contains a mutation in the DNA code of a gene called KRAS, then the medicines cetuximab (Erbitux) and panitumomab (Vectibix) will not be used because they will not add benefit to chemotherapy.

The extent and aggressiveness of the cancer. A rapidly growing, life-threatening cancer usually requires more intensive therapy than may be required to control a less threatening cancer.

The age and medical condition of the patient. These factors help guide the oncologist to choose treatments that the patient can tolerate physically without excessive toxicity.

The wishes of the patient. This is paramount in any treatment decision. Given a choice of treatments, oncologists will recommend those most in keeping with the patient's needs: for example, chemotherapy that spares hair is given when possible to those for whom hair loss is anathema. It is vital that the patient and oncologist have open communication and a good rapport so that the patient can accurately convey how much he or she wants to fight and what type of side effects he or she is willing to tolerate. Good communication ensures that patients feel their doctor understands them and what they are about as people and cancer patients.

The availability of a clinical trial. Cancers that are not routinely curable demand that we try to do better. It is only by conducting research studies that better cancer treatments will be found. The National Institutes of Health and National Cancer Institute are expanding their efforts to make clinical trials available to all cancer patients (www

.clinicaltrials.gov). All oncologists need to provide their patients with access to new therapies; cancer patients, for their part, need to consider participating in these studies both for their own benefit and for the greater good.

Once a treatment is chosen, the duration of therapy is decided upon so that the patient knows what to expect. Treatment may be for a specified time (for example, six cycles of chemotherapy) or open-ended: a treatment is continued as long as it is well tolerated and deemed to be working.

Evaluation of the cancer by CT scans or other tests may be performed at regular intervals during treatment (for example, after every two to three cycles) to make certain the treatment is working. On completion of therapy, a break is given in order to allow the patient's body (and psyche) to recover. Thereafter, regular follow-up examinations and imaging studies may be employed to track the condition of the patient and status of the disease. Treatments are resumed if the cancer regrows; the six factors are again employed to guide the choice of second-line therapy and beyond.

> *A metastatic cancer may be contained over time through the sequential use of one therapy after another.*

The treatment of many forms of metastatic cancer (such as those of the breast, colon, prostate, and lung) has become continuous: treatments are administered at regular intervals (often weekly or every other week) until they are deemed ineffective or the patient needs a break. If treatment is working after several months on therapy but side effects are accumulating or blood counts remain low, then breaks in treatment may be given. If several drugs are being used successfully, the harshest one may be halted for a period of time; this approach is being tested on numerous cancers.

Should the cancer enter a complete remission, treatment may be halted and the patient closely monitored, depending on the comfort levels of both patient and physician. Some patients feel uneasy without treatment, whereas others can't wait to put therapy out of their minds for awhile. Typically, a patient and his or her oncologist will engage in a give and take regarding the merits and toxicities of continuing treatment beyond a certain point. The oncologist should initiate and guide these discussions.

Although I have said that oncologists love data, there is little data regarding stopping points for chronic cancer treatments that are working. Common practice patterns have emerged, with a tendency to continue treatment, as outlined above.

THE BOND BETWEEN PATIENT AND PHYSICIAN IS TIGHT

The ability to care for patients with metastatic cancer so that they can continue to function in their daily lives takes great clinical skill and is as much an art as a science. Research techniques such as genomic profiling of cancer (discussed in chapter 3) will eventually enable oncologists to select "the right treatment for the right cancer." But nothing will replace good old-fashioned doctoring, the ability to sense and know when a treatment is or is not helping.

Patients with metastatic cancers see their oncologists often. Frequent communication enables physicians to get to know their patients, to know when they have a bounce to their step and feel well or if they appear to have lost a step and are ill (or depressed). As in the case I described earlier of Patrick the painter, I know whenever he says that he is not painting that either the cancer is getting worse or the treatment is getting the better of him. Either way, something different needs to be done.

Many patients put up a good front in the presence of their oncologists. They do so mainly out of fear that an admission of sickness might indicate that the cancer is growing but also to avoid appearing "weak"; they want to prove that they can "take it." Because even the most sensitive physician is not a mind reader, if you are a patient, I encourage you to be honest and direct with your oncologist about how you are feeling so that you can receive the treatments most helpful to your situation.

Cancer in the Older Individual

The challenge in caring for people with advanced cancer is perhaps tested most acutely when elderly and especially extremely old people get cancer. A fine line must be walked between the benefits of treatment to prolong life or control cancer-related symptoms and the ease with which treatments provoke side effects.

Aging diminishes the capacity of a number of organs in the body that affect cancer treatment, including: the bone marrow and the ability of blood counts to withstand chemotherapy; the liver and the ability to metabolize drugs; the kidney and the ability to eliminate drugs; and the brain and the ability to remember complex medication schedules. Beyond the purely physical, many older individuals have lost a spouse or suffer from loneliness and a predisposition to depression. At a time of life when greater support is needed, often less support exists.

But life is full of the unexpected, and sometimes good can come from bad. The interaction of an older cancer patient with a vibrant cancer center can get that person beyond his or her four walls into a lively and welcoming place where "somebody knows your name." With laughter, art workshops, support groups in which to socialize, and even snacks, the importance of community cancer centers in treating the older patient (or anyone) cannot be overstated.

Researchers are trying to develop cancer-specific geriatric assessment tools to help oncologists better judge which treatments an older patient can tolerate. When older people become cancer patients, they are especially wary of taking treatments that may not help them live substantially longer but may make them ill during their remaining days. Until we can predict how well an individual will tolerate cancer treatments, physicians will have to use their powers of perception and clinical judgment or rely on the assessments of a spouse: "Look at him. He's eighty-six and looks great. He mows the lawn, walks a mile every day, and eats me out of house and home. God bless him!"

A vignette: Catherine, an extraordinary eighty-four-year-old woman, legally blind, published nonfiction author, beloved mother and grandmother, came to see me after being diagnosed with stage IV lung cancer. The cancer was detected after severe back pain led her to see her doctor. CT scans showed that the culprit was a tumor pressing on her spinal cord. Catherine had once been a smoker, and a chest CT scan found the primary lung cancer. Biopsy confirmed the diagnosis. She agreed to meet with an oncologist, though she "did not expect much to come of it."

At our first meeting, Catherine made it clear that she was realistic about her condition and was not afraid of death. Yet, she said, she would like to live without pain and "wouldn't mind living longer. I do have a book in the works and would love to finish it."

The initial strategy was to avoid anticancer drug treatments (and their side effects) and focus on the symptoms the cancer was causing. If the cancer grew slowly, such a strategy could maintain her quality of life for some time. Radiation treatments to the tumor on her spine greatly improved her pain. She began monthly infusions of Zometa to prevent bone fractures and weekly injections of Procrit to improve her anemia (in this case caused by the cancer) and energy level.

Two months later Catherine developed shoulder pain and weakness, signs that the cancer was progressing. Pain medication was prescribed. She and I discussed that although drug treatments could not cure the cancer, they might slow its growth. Despite her age, there were therapies that, without causing major side effects, might improve how she felt and possibly prolong her life. If a treatment was tried, it could always be stopped. With understandable hesitation, Catherine agreed to try.

We started with a targeted therapy in the hopes of avoiding significant side effects, but it made Catherine feel weak. The dose was lowered and the pill continued for a month. Her cancer symptoms did not improve, so the treatment was abandoned. She agreed to try an intravenous chemotherapy drug given once a week that, to her surprise, did not make her sick at all; in fact, she felt better than when taking the non-chemo pill. Unfortunately, this treatment also proved ineffective.

Fatigue and pain were gradually increasing, but Catherine was still strong enough to make office visits and live independently. I explained that her symptoms would not improve unless we gained some control over the cancer. We openly and thoroughly discussed all her options, including stopping cancer treatments and choosing hospice. Becoming resigned to losing her battle with cancer soon, she admitted that she intended to turn down any book contract she was offered rather than commit to an obligation she could not fulfill.

Sensing that I had one last opportunity to help her, I offered another chemotherapy drug that, if given at a lowered dose, would not cause debilitating side effects or hair loss (this was important to her). After two weekly injections, she appeared stronger, did not rely on her cane as much, and sat in my office smiling. "I feel really well. I have no pain and I want to do things," she said. "I have no idea what this means. I'm actually shocked. Is this the end of the beginning or the beginning of the end?"

Two months later, Catherine began an office visit by stating, "I have bad news." I was put off-balance: "You have bad news for me? What is it? I thought things were going well?" Her reply: "I signed a book contract." I started howling and said, "That's fantastic, congratulations!" She replied somewhat sheepishly, "I hated to tell you. The whole process is so unfair" (she was aware of my difficulties as a first-time author in getting this book published). She then sat up energetically, looked me in the eye, and said, "Okay. Now you have to make me live forever."

The Role of Surgery in Metastatic Cancer

If a stage IV cancer forms metastases in several regions of the body, then surgery will play a limited role because surgeons cannot remove large portions of the lungs, brain, and bones in an effort to eradicate tumors in these locations. The focus is, by necessity, on treatments that attack the cancer throughout the body—namely, drugs.

Yet surgery can play a pivotal role leading to the long-term survival of some individuals with stage IV cancer. Some cancers form metastases that are confined to one organ, called "isolated metastases." This situation may be encountered at diagnosis or when a cancer relapses some time after its initial treatment. The target organs tend to be the brain, liver, or lung, and the approach to removing metastases in each region is different.

Surgical removal of isolated metastases is usually performed only if the operation can remove all visible areas of the disease; removal of only some of the cancer deposits in an organ will not lead to the goal of cure or long-term cancer control. When the brain is affected by one or two isolated metastases, then surgery is often feasible; this may be followed by radiation, depending on the situation. When the lungs are affected by isolated metastases, then surgery to remove the tumors may be performed even if there are numerous metastases. The lung is typically affected by isolated metastases from cancers originating in the colon and rectum, kidney, and testes, as well as from some types of sarcoma. Chemotherapy may be given before surgery to shrink the tumors and is often given afterward to prevent new tumors from growing.

Isolated metastases to the liver are mainly associated with cancers of the colon and rectum. In years past, surgeons would remove only three or fewer metastases contained in a limited part of the liver. Today, experienced liver surgeons can remove up to 80 percent of the liver to render the patient cancer-free, regardless of the number or size of the cancer deposits! Amazingly, the liver regenerates itself in a matter of weeks. Chemotherapy is often given before and after this type of surgery.

Several other techniques are used to treat cancer affecting the liver: (1) hepatic artery infusion, in which chemotherapy is instilled directly into the liver through an implanted pump; (2) chemoembolization, in which an interventional radiologist infuses chemotherapy and a substance that chokes off the blood supply to tumors (this technique is used mostly for neuroendocrine cancers and primary liver cancer); (3) cryotherapy, in which tumors are destroyed by freezing; and (4) radiofrequency ablation, in which tumors are destroyed by heat.

Rather than forming a limited number of metastases, however, most stage IV cancers form numerous cancer deposits located in various parts of the body. For example, a person who undergoes colonoscopy and is found to have a colon cancer would have a CT scan of the chest and abdomen as part of the staging workup. If numerous cancer growths are found in both the liver and the lungs, the metastases could not be removed to render the patient cancer-free. Still, it would be natural to ask, "Shouldn't the cancer in the colon be taken out even if the metastases cannot be surgically removed?"

In regard to any newly diagnosed metastatic cancer, it is common to ask, "Isn't there value in removing a primary tumor despite the presence of metastases?" Aside from the natural desire to rid the body of as much cancer as possible, I have heard two main reasons for patients asking about this surgery: Is the main tumor somehow supporting the growth of distant metastases in some way, like a queen bee sustaining her hive? And won't the main tumor continue to seed the body with metastases if it is not removed?

The answer to the second question is more straightforward: although the main tumor can remain a source of ongoing metastasis, drug treatments are preferred over surgery because they will silence this process as well as treat the cancer throughout the body. Removing the primary is unlikely to improve the chances for cure and would only delay the administration of the required chemotherapy. Therefore, despite the natural inclination to remove the primary, it is not routinely done as the initial treatment.

The first question is more complicated but also more fascinating. There are animal models of human cancer (for example, human lung cancer cells capable of growing in a mouse) in which removal of the primary tumor results in rapid growth of distant metastases. These models were intensively studied, and it was determined that a substance generated by the primary tumor travels through the bloodstream to put the brakes on growth of metastases found elsewhere in the body (that is, the primary cancer inhibits growth of its own metastases). Dr. Judah Folkman isolated the first such compound and discovered that it prevented metastases from growing by blocking their ability to form a blood supply (called angiogenesis inhibitor therapy). He named the compound angiostatin, and it lit a fire in the world of cancer drug development. Today, nearly forty angiogenesis inhibitor compounds are under study for the treatment of cancer. Folkman's discoveries have revolutionized how we think of and treat cancer.

In the real world, cancer does not often behave the same in a mouse as it does in a human. In fact, the ability of a primary tumor to slow the growth of its own metastases is *not* a common finding in humans; if a primary needs to come out, then it should be taken out without hesitation (an example would be a large tumor in the colon that was causing complete obstruction). The only situation in which removal of a primary tumor has been conclusively demonstrated to have an effect on survival is in metastatic kidney cancer. But this effect is a positive one: among patients with metastatic kidney cancer treated with interferon, those who first undergo removal of the primary cancer (and involved kidney) live longer than those in whom the primary tumor is left in place.

The Role of Radiation Therapy in Metastatic Cancer

When cancer is present in more than one region of the body, radiation treatments cannot eradicate it, but they can improve symptoms caused by tumors in specific areas. Radiation therapy can be given to virtually any part of the body. Two of the most common uses of radiation in the treatment of metastatic cancer are discussed below.

Radiation therapy is the mainstay of treatment for cancer metastases affecting the brain. In this situation, whole brain radiation therapy (WBRT) is typically given daily, five days a week, for two or more weeks. A steroid medication called dexamethasone (Decadron) is usually prescribed during treatment to decrease the swelling that typically surrounds metastases and which may worsen during radiation. Typical side effects of WBRT include reversible hair loss (the hair takes a good number of months to return), temporary scalp irritation, and mild weakness. Memory impairment and other neurological side effects are uncommon. Overall, WBRT is surprisingly well tolerated and generally does not impair the patient's functional level during treatment. As with all cancer therapies, if the cancer is causing symptoms (brain metastases may cause headaches, imbalance, nausea, weakness, and specific neurologic impairment), then the therapy will greatly improve a person's condition.

If isolated brain metastases (usually no more than three) are present and surgery is best avoided, then stereotactic radiosurgery (a form of radiation, not surgery) can be performed. This focuses high-intensity beams on a small region of the brain. WBRT may be used before or after this procedure in an effort to prevent new brain lesions from developing in regions outside the stereotactic field. The radiation oncologist and neurosurgeon will coordinate the best plan of attack on brain metastases. The use of chemotherapy and targeted therapies to improve the effectiveness of radiation against brain metastases is being tested.

Individual areas of cancer metastases in the bones and around the spinal cord may also be treated with radiation therapy, especially if they are causing pain, difficulty walking, or specific neurological symptoms. Patients with bone metastases may also receive regular infusions of a bone-strengthening drug, such as zoledronic acid (Zometa) or pamidronate (Aredia), which decrease the risk of fracture caused by the cancer.

It is critical to seek consultation and care with a medical oncologist before beginning radiation treatments for a cancer that has metastasized (unless treatment is urgent) so that the sequencing of radiation with other treatments that may be needed (such as chemotherapy) can be optimally planned. In many treatment centers, radiation oncologists and medical oncologists are within walking distance of one another, which facilitates good and timely communication about the treatment plan for their patients; the multidisciplinary care of cancer patients is also coordinated at regularly scheduled hospital tumor boards.

In summary, the appropriate treatment of any cancer is dictated by specific aspects of the cancer as well as the health and preferences of the patient. Cancer treatments given with the intent and possibility of cure (adjuvant and neoadjuvant therapies, some metastatic cancers) should be given at the recommended doses; they are administered over a finite period. On the other hand, there is more flexibility in the administration of treatments for metastatic (chronic) cancers: the treatment period is indefinite and may be off and on for the remainder of a person's life. As tremendous advances in science bear fruit in the everyday treatment of people with cancer, survival will continue to improve and many more people will be living with the disease.

We must always keep in mind, however, that the goal of treatment in these situations is not to extend one's suffering but rather to improve one's quality of life and diminish cancer-related symptoms; when this occurs, enhanced survival is sure to follow.

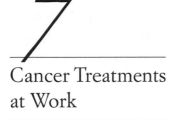

7

Cancer Treatments
at Work

At the end of a hectic day not long ago, I was asked to consult on an urgent case: an eighty-eight-year-old hospitalized patient who was in a coma. The referring doctor, a caring physician, stated bluntly, "He's very sick and close to death. The scans show widespread cancer, though we haven't done a biopsy. Given his age, I think the best way to proceed is hospice, and I've recommended this to his sons. They're very realistic but want to meet with an oncologist for closure."

The patient, Abe, was a retired dentist who had been living with his wife in another state. For some time he had been experiencing fevers, weight loss, and progressive weakness. But because his wife had Alzheimer's disease and he looked after her, he neglected his own declining health. The couple's sons had recently visited them and immediately insisted that their parents return home for medical care. By the time Abe was examined by a physician, he required hospitalization; he was too weak to walk, was becoming confused, and soon after lost consciousness.

I encountered a long, gaunt, handsome man in a hospital bed; he had a shock of white hair and few wrinkles, appearing younger than his age.

His temperature was 103 degrees and he was clammy to the touch. He did not open his eyes when I called his name and only moaned when I shook him. CT scans to locate a source of fever had revealed a tumor the size of a volleyball in his abdomen, smaller tumors in his chest, and widespread involvement of the bones. The situation was grim.

According to his sons, Abe had been alert and clear thinking until the current illness. They wanted to know whether there was any chance he could improve and whether it was worthwhile to pursue a biopsy to determine the type of cancer he had. I told them that it probably wasn't, adding that I rarely said this. Given his age, debilitated condition, and widespread malignancy, even a very treatable cancer such as lymphoma would probably not turn around in time. The chances of success were low.

And how would we define success? If we could shrink the cancer but Abe remained in a coma, would we have helped him? What if treatments only prolonged his suffering? Certainly the case could be made for being humane and letting him pass, since he was so close. They acknowledged all of this and said they would confer and get back to me with their decision.

Not long after, they called. "Dad was always a fighter and tough as nails. He would want to know what he had. And he would want to try to fight. We can't let him go without at least knowing what he has. That would not be honoring the way he lived his life, the way he taught us to be. So let's do the biopsy, let's go for it." I replied, "Fine, let's do it. But we have to act quickly. I want the biopsy done this afternoon so we can have a result by tomorrow."

The diagnosis was large cell lymphoma. "I can't predict whether the cancer will respond to treatment or if he'll wake up," I told them, "but he probably won't experience severe side effects from the recommended chemotherapy. If we're going to try, let's do it right and give him every chance." Again they conferred and said that they would get back to me. I got the call: "Fire away." We administered CHOP-Rixutan therapy and hoped for the best.

I saw Abe the next morning on my rounds, and his fever was down, attributable to the steroid medication he received as part of the treatment. He looked more comfortable but was still unresponsive. His sons milled around the halls while his wife sat by his side, quiet and pensive. I returned the next day to find no change. I saw him on the third, fourth, fifth, and sixth days following treatment. He lay motionless in the bed, with no signs of improvement. All I could do was counsel his family.

On the seventh morning, I made my rounds early. The hospital was quiet, and Abe was alone in his room. I stood at his bedside and performed my usual examination. Out of habit, I called his name, not expecting a response. There was none. But as I turned to leave, he sprang bolt upright, opened crystal-clear blue eyes, and blurted out emphatically as he tapped on his right temple, "My name is Abe, and I have all my marbles!" I was flabbergasted. He continued and became choked up, "Thank you, doctor, thank you for all you've done."

I was floored, tongue-tied, and choked up, too. "Well . . . I can see that you do . . . have all your marbles! You are so welcome!"

Abe received additional treatments and achieved a remission of his cancer. He enjoyed more time with his family and actually survived his wife; he died not long after she did of causes unrelated to cancer.

I relate this story to illustrate the sometimes dramatic results that can be obtained with effective chemotherapy.

A New Era of Hope

Cancer was recognized thousands of years ago, but only recently have we felt comfortable mentioning "the C word" and discussing this disease openly. The pink ribbon and the yellow LIVESTRONG wristband are symbols recognized the world over and represent our collective hope for the conquest of cancer. We are more comfortable talking about cancer because of the many improvements in treatment that have come about in the past forty years. Almost everybody knows somebody who is a survivor. Advances are announced frequently in the news. Surgery is becoming less invasive, radiation therapy more pinpointed and intense. Research is yielding an array of promising new drugs. Although we have far to go in reaching our goals for many cancers, we are indeed living in a new era of hope in which the chances of surviving even advanced cancer improve every year.

The medicines that underlie the revolution in the management of cancer are the focus of this chapter. Oncologists currently have at their disposal approximately one hundred individual drugs and many drug combinations to treat cancer. Several hundred new medicines and immune treatments are being developed and tested in clinical trials. Thousands more are undoubtedly being hatched in the fertile brains of today's cancer researchers. The treatment targets are not just the cancer cells but also the surrounding normal tissues that support them.

Cancer-fighting drugs can be classified into three broad categories:

1. Chemotherapy
2. Targeted therapies
3. Hormone therapies

(Immune therapies such as vaccines and cell-based therapies are not yet standard treatment, although there is great hope for their success. Interferon and interleukin are approved but are not discussed in detail here. Some targeted therapies also activate the immune system to fight cancer, as discussed below.)

In this chapter, I explain how cancer-fighting drugs work, as well as how radiation therapy works. The accompanying images enable you to visualize cancer being eradicated by these treatments. If you are a cancer patient, ask your oncologist which types of medicines you are receiving (many patients receive more than one type), and go to those sections to fix an image in your "mind's eye" of what those treatments are doing to your cancer. Visualizing cancer being rubbed out and the body healing will be empowering and give you a greater sense of control over the disease.

Examples of cancer-fighting medicines are given throughout this chapter. Appendix 1 contains a more complete listing of these medicines and classifies them based on how they work, as described below.

Targeting the Lifelines of Cancer

Whether we are considering chemotherapy, targeted therapies, or hormone therapies, most cancer-fighting medicines converge on the lifelines of a cancer cell—namely, its communications network.

Like the normal cells from which they are derived, cancer cells rely heavily on their ability to communicate in order to function. They send and receive signals from nearby cancer cells as well as from surrounding healthy cells in order to survive and grow. Our cells have evolved a highly specialized communications network that is made up of a large and complex network of interacting molecules: signals dart around furiously as they might on a computer chip. Cancer cells co-opt critical nodes on this chip in the form of molecules that increase the signals to grow, spread, and resist death (see chapter 1). As scientists identify these crucial molecules, drugs can be designed to block their function and shut down a line of communication. If this line is vital, the cancer cell may implode and die.

Both normal and cancer cells are protected from the "outside world" by a layer of fat called the lipid membrane. This membrane separates the watery environment of the inside of a cell from the rest of the body. Embedded within the lipid shield are tiny proteins called receptors that often span its width (see fig. 15). Many millions of receptors on the cell surface function like antennae, picking up signals from the surrounding environment and transmitting them to the inner world of the cell on the other side of the lipid layer. Each type of receptor can be stimulated by only one or a few molecules, much as a lock can be opened by only one key.

Once a surface receptor becomes activated, it initiates a cascade of signals (think of falling dominoes) that travel through the cell to reach the destination, the DNA. These communications transmissions are a form of chemical energy that is passed like a baton in a relay race from one signaling molecule to the next. Ultimately, the final molecule in the relay heads to the DNA finish line, where it latches onto the double helix and modifies what DNA directs the cell to do; DNA responds by sending out new commands that ramify back throughout the cell. The DNA may signal the cell to duplicate itself to increase the size of a tumor, spread to a new location to form a metastasis, or stay alive despite the body's effort to eradicate it. The goal of cancer treatments is to disrupt this flow of information in the cancer cell, ultimately causing it to die.

The three main components of the cancer communications system can be thought of as residing at different "levels" of a cancer cell: surface receptors at the outer layer, internal signaling molecules on the inside, and DNA embedded in the deepest part of a cell. Each component serves as a target for modern-day cancer-fighting drugs:

- Chemotherapy blocks DNA from functioning properly.
- Targeted therapies block surface receptors and/or signaling molecules from communicating their signals.
- Hormone therapies prevent estrogen or testosterone from generating growth signals in the cancer cell.

Each type of therapy works in a specific way to disrupt cell communication. Even though only one type carries the name "targeted," each does seek out and attach to particular targets in the cell; even chemotherapy drugs attack specific regions of the DNA. Whereas targeted therapies are designed to block known targets, many chemotherapy drugs were originally discovered based primarily on their cancer-fighting properties before their targets in the cell were identified. It is because the targets of chemotherapy are so large (a cell's entire DNA) and exist in nearly every cell of the body that chemotherapy tends to cause more side effects than targeted therapies.

Because many genetic derangements affect most cancers, often several pathways in the communications network must be disrupted to force a cancer cell to shut down. Accordingly, many patients are being treated with chemotherapy plus one or more targeted therapies to achieve a result superior to either type of therapy alone. As always, the most appropriate therapy depends on the specific cancer, the treatments that have already been used, and the medical condition of the patient.

Chemotherapy

Chemotherapy drugs represent a diverse collection of chemicals that have been proven effective in treating cancer. Each type of cancer responds to different chemotherapy drugs, although some drugs can be effective against many cancers. More than half of all chemotherapy drugs come from nature or are derivatives of natural compounds. For example, doxorubicin (Adriamycin) is made by a fungus, paclitaxel (Taxol) and docetaxel (Taxotere) come from the Pacific yew tree, and irinotecan (Camptosar) was isolated from a Chinese ornamental plant.

These drugs were found mainly through an extensive and ongoing effort of the National Cancer Institute to screen compounds made by plants, bacteria, fungi, and marine life for their cancer-fighting properties. A number of other chemotherapies have been "rationally" constructed by scientists to interfere with known mechanisms of cell growth. Still others have been discovered by serendipity.

Most chemotherapy drugs work by damaging DNA. They do so through a variety of mechanisms too complex to discuss here. Examples include doxorubicin, carboplatin, cisplatin, oxaliplatin, Cytoxan, 5-FU, fludarabine (Fludara), gemcitabine (Gemzar), and capecitabine (Xeloda). For a more complete list, see appendix 1.

Mainly, the drugs chemically attack DNA, like metal to a magnet, causing the double helix to break; they may also interfere with the cell's DNA repair machinery, leading to further fragmentation of the genetic code. If the DNA, the cell's molecular brain trust, sustains extensive damage, then the cell commits suicide or undergoes apoptosis (discussed in chapter 1). The action of chemotherapy inside a cancer cell is illustrated in figure 13.

Some chemotherapy drugs do not affect DNA but instead target a different cell structure called microtubules to prevent a cell from multiplying, as I explain next.

One of the most important signals that DNA communicates is for a cell to divide or multiply (by a process called mitosis). This is the process by which one cell becomes two; it is the grist for the mill of cancer

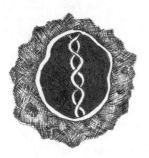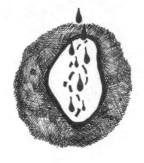

Fig. 13. *Chemotherapy attacking cancer*
A cancer cell dies when its DNA is attacked by chemotherapy. Illustration
© Gale V. Parsons.

growth. For this to occur, the DNA duplicates itself to form two copies; each copy goes to the opposite ends of the cell. Next, the cell splits down the middle, and two newly minted cells pinch apart from each other; an analogy would be the twisting of a long balloon to make two halves, which magically separate and seal at their ends to make two balloons. Normal cell division is shown in figure 14A.

This complicated process is dependent on a cell component called microtubules, long fibers that push the DNA to opposite poles of a cell and pull the two newly forming cells apart. Drugs like paclitaxel (Taxol) and docetaxel (Taxotere) prevent the push and pull of the microtubules and freeze the cell in place; the result is cancer cell death, as shown in figure 14B. Other drugs in this class are indicated in appendix 1.

The ability of chemotherapy drugs to preferentially kill cancer cells rather than normal cells rests with the fact that more cells are dividing in a cancerous tumor than in the other tissues of the body. As a result, cancer DNA and microtubules are more susceptible to chemotherapy-induced damage. For example, chemotherapy given for cancer that has spread to the lungs or liver will affect the cancer there but not likely damage the surrounding lungs or liver; in fact, normal organ function may improve if the damaging effects of the cancer are diminished.

Chemotherapy drugs may work in other ways to eliminate cancer cells. One way is by reducing the blood flow to a tumor (called angio-

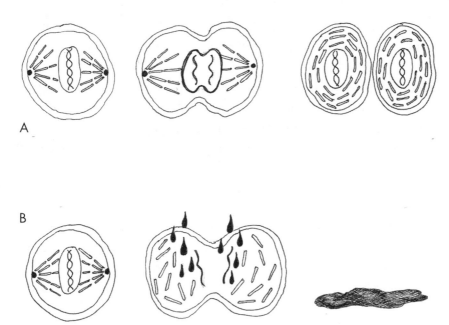

Fig. 14. *Chemotherapy blocking cancer cell duplication*
A cancer cell is shown dividing into two cells (A); this process is dependent on spindle shaped structures called microtubules. When microtubules are attacked by certain chemotherapy drugs, such as Taxol and Taxotere, the cell cannot divide but rather dies (B). Illustration © Gale V. Parsons.

genesis inhibition, discussed below). This effect is associated with frequently administered drugs, such as daily pills or weekly intravenous injections. Blood flow to the tumor is reduced when the blood vessel–forming cells that feed it are killed; like cancer cells, these cells are also busy multiplying, building a blood supply for the cancer.

THE MODERN ERA OF CHEMOTHERAPY

Talking about chemotherapy is like talking about the weather: on any given day, in any part of the world, there can be perfect calm or there may be a blizzard.

When discussing the side effects of chemotherapy, just as when discussing the weather, it is important to avoid generalizations and not lump all chemotherapy together. The specific drugs, doses, and schedules in which chemotherapy is given as well as the patient's constitution determine how well it is tolerated. Whereas some chemotherapy regimens are very hard on the body, others are compatible with normal routines. Before receiving chemotherapy, patients are usually given fact sheets describing the possible (likely and less likely) side effects of each medicine as well as the opportunity to meet with an oncology nurse to talk about what to expect.

Fears about chemotherapy drugs can cause great anxiety among those about to undergo treatment. A great deal of *mis*information exists about their side effects. Some of this is a holdover from days long gone when cancer patients receiving chemotherapy frequently experienced nausea and vomiting as well as a greatly diminished ability to prevent certain infections. We are now in the modern era of chemotherapy, in which many of the most severe side effects have been greatly improved by a host of medications.

In the section below, my intent is not to minimize the serious side effects that chemotherapy can sometimes cause and about which there is ample information. My goal is to clarify the misconceptions about chemotherapy that I frequently hear from new patients in my oncology practice.

If you are undergoing chemotherapy treatments, I recommend reading the pamphlet *Chemotherapy and You,* available free from the National Cancer Institute (1-800-4-CANCER). It contains helpful information on managing the side effects of chemotherapy.

MYTHS AND FACTS ABOUT CHEMOTHERAPY

Myth: Chemotherapy always causes nausea and vomiting.

Fact: If you are about to receive chemotherapy, visit the infusion suite where your treatment will be administered. Look around. You will see other patients receiving intravenous medications. Some will be reading, others listening to music or having a conversation. You will even see many of them eating. But you will probably not see anyone vomiting.

When a cancer patient sits down to receive chemotherapy, the first medications the oncology nurse will hang on the IV pole are not the cancer-fighting drugs but rather premedications or "premeds." Premeds include antinausea and other medications that reduce the risk of side effects. Advances in new medicines that prevent nausea and vomiting have dramatically improved the tolerability of chemotherapy. As a result, the chemotherapy session is often anticlimactic, even uneventful.

Once at home, nausea may or may not occur. It might begin the night of treatment or the next day. If nausea does occur, then antinausea medications should be taken as directed by your oncology doctor or nurse. Before you begin chemotherapy, make sure your doctor gives you a prescription for one (or more) of these medicines in case you need them; better to have them on hand and unused than having to call for them at 3:00 am. If they are not sufficient, call your doctor's office at any time of the day or night and speak to the oncologist on call for help.

The chances that nausea and vomiting will occur depend on the type of chemotherapy drugs administered and on the individual; every person will react differently. Your oncology team will tell you whether the drugs you will receive are associated with a low, intermediate, or high risk of nausea. Medications and other techniques to prevent the symptoms (such as sea bands, eating ginger, and smelling lemons) will be recommended accordingly. If after the first chemotherapy session you experience excessive nausea and/or vomiting, a change in antinausea medication will be prescribed to improve the situation for the next treatment.

Overall, most patients experience only mild nausea after chemotherapy. For some, nausea may last for one or a few days and then disappear. Others find that they always have a low level of nausea while undergoing therapy that does not prevent them from eating; still others come to expect "one good puke" the morning after that rights their systems. Whichever pattern you may experience, the management of this miserable side effect is infinitely better than it was a decade ago.

Myth: Chemotherapy wreaks havoc on the immune system.

Fact: This fear relates to the fact that *some* (but not all) chemotherapy drugs can lower the white blood cell (WBC) count and, consequently, the body's ability to fight certain infections. The specific kind of WBC that protects against bacterial infections is called a neutrophil; a low neutrophil count is called neutropenia.

A normal neutrophil count is above 1,800 in Caucasians and 1,400 in African Americans. The risk of infection rises substantially when the neutrophil count is less than 1,000 and especially under 500. Infection is often heralded by a fever called neutropenic fever. This can be life threatening when not addressed in a timely manner.

If you are receiving chemotherapy and you experience a fever (100.4 degrees or above), contact your oncologist right away, even if it is the middle of the night. Do not *take fever-reducing medicines on your own and try to sleep it off.*

Owing to major advancements in science, medications now exist to bolster a person's WBC and neutrophils; they have dramatically reduced the risk of severe infections experienced by cancer patients. They include: filgrastim (Neupogen), sargramostatin (Leukine), and pegfilgrastim (Neulasta, a longer-acting Neupogen), which are administered as subcutaneous injections. These "drugs" are actually natural chemicals made by our bodies to stimulate bone marrow function.

Surprisingly, most of the infections that affect the neutropenic cancer patient come from the body; the *E. coli* and other bacteria that normally reside in the intestinal tract are a major source. Other sources of infection may be rotten teeth, breaks in the skin, or catheters placed for the purpose of receiving chemotherapy.

Oncologists may prescribe a WBC growth factor in two ways: (1) to *treat* neutropenia (and especially neutropenic fever) when it occurs after cancer treatments; or (2) to *prevent* neutropenia through administration of the medication on the day or days following chemotherapy.

Only some patients undergoing chemotherapy will require the use of a WBC growth factor. Their need depends on the intensity of the cancer treatment as well as on aspects of their condition and history. Patients who have had chemotherapy or radiation therapy in the past, those with low blood counts before starting chemotherapy (for reasons their doctor should investigate), and the elderly are more prone to develop neutropenia from chemotherapy.

It is important to realize that WBC growth factors do not eliminate neutropenia and the risk of infection; despite their use, strong chemotherapy will still cause neutropenia. Rather, by minimizing the duration or number of days of neutropenia, WBC growth factors limit the time during which a patient is most susceptible to infection.

Although there will always be a risk of infection with chemotherapy, the proper use of WBC growth factors and antibiotics, along with the oncology team's close attention to the patient's condition, has made "a wreck of the immune system" a thing of the past.

Myth: Chemotherapy always causes baldness.

Fact: Some but not all chemotherapy drugs cause significant hair loss. Science has not found a way to prevent this side effect. The hair will grow back, usually beginning about four to six weeks after the completion of therapy. In some cases, hair may regrow while a patient is receiving the chemotherapy that made it fall out in the first place (this does not mean that the chemotherapy is no longer working). The first growth is like peach fuzz, eventually resulting in a wavy, soft new head of hair (sorry, but gray hair will not come back as dark hair). In contrast, some chemotherapy drugs may only cause hair thinning, and others will have little effect on hair growth.

Many patients find it best to prepare for possible or expected hair loss by visiting a wigmaker before their hair falls out and by cutting their hair short once chemotherapy has started; they should carry a prescription for a "cranial prosthesis" so that the cost is covered by insurance. Any cancer center is clearly full of individuals (patients and staff) who are familiar with this process and able to provide excellent advice.

Myth: Chemotherapy causes weakness and an inability to carry out normal activities.

Fact: If you are experiencing symptoms from cancer, then effective chemotherapy will make you feel better, not worse. Only when the cancer is treated can the body heal.

For any cancer patient, however, chemotherapy may certainly contribute to weakness. The longer treatments go on, the more likely it is that fatigue will be a part of a patient's life. But this fatigue is usually not debilitating. Most patients undergoing chemotherapy will be able to function in their lives with some modifications. Parents may need help at home; workers may need to cut back their hours or take time off to complete treatment; travel is often minimized. The types of treatments and the patient's physical condition and age are again critical determinants of the severity of fatigue.

Anemia, or a low red blood count, is one reason for weakness. Some cancers suppress bone marrow activity, which can lead to anemia before chemotherapy starts. Blood levels of folic acid, vitamin B12, and iron should also be checked; the oncologist may need to consider unrelated bone marrow disorders if severe anemia is present and unexplained. When chemotherapy causes anemia, it is not immediate but rather emerges after two or three cycles of treatment. Chemotherapy may lower red blood production just as it does white blood cell production. In such cases, injections of red blood cell (RBC) growth factors, called erythropoietin (Procrit) or darbopoietin (Aranesp), are administered. Erythropoietin is the hormone that our kidneys normally make to stimulate the bone marrow to generate red blood; all patients receiving dialysis for kidney failure receive these medications.

Other factors that may contribute to weakness include insufficient rest, inadequate nutrition, depression, anxiety, stress, and psychological distress caused by what cancer is doing to the patient's life. I encourage every cancer patient to discuss these issues with his or her oncologist and to seek help in addressing them with professionals such as clinical social workers and psychiatrists. There is no value in suffering through cancer and its treatments; the short-term use of medications or psychological counseling can do a world of good.

Myth: Chemotherapy destroys good cells along with the bad.

Fact: Each chemotherapy drug has a number of well-established side effects that oncologists discuss with their patients before treatment. Most centers provide patients with chemotherapy fact cards or sheets that describe common and less common side effects caused by the drugs to be used. Similar to common medications filled by prescription, the lists of possible side effects from a chemotherapy drug are long (and often frightening). And like any other medication, only a fraction of the listed side effects will occur; the intensity of each side effect will also vary from person to person.

Just as only certain chemotherapy drugs cause significant nausea, hair loss, or fatigue, some drugs are associated with the potential to cause damage to the heart, lungs, kidneys, reproductive organs, or other organs. This damage, or decline in function, may be temporary or long lasting. It may be mild (not noticed by the patient) or "clinically significant," which means that the problem is affecting the patient's ability to function normally. In order to monitor "the rest of the body" and not just the cancer, vital organ function is tested at regular intervals during cancer treatment and for many years after treatment has finished (see chapter 8 regarding care of the cancer survivor).

It should be noted that if a patient has some impairment of vital organ function before beginning treatment (such as kidney insufficiency or congestive heart failure), then some chemotherapy drugs will be administered in reduced doses and others will be avoided.

Even for those chemotherapy drugs associated with damage to a particular organ, the damage is usually avoided if precautions are taken. For example, when the drug cisplatin (Platinol) was introduced in the 1960s, its anticancer activity was remarkable, but it also caused kidney failure in the first studies and was nearly abandoned. Fortunately, it was shown that if extra fluids were given intravenously along with the drug, kidney failure could be averted. Cisplatin went on to cure testicular cancer and is used safely today in a variety of cancers. Patients receiving cisplatin today are told to drink fluids liberally before and for twenty-four hours after administration.

As part of the education process before chemotherapy, cancer patients will be informed of any possible organ damage from the drugs

173

they will receive and any precautions that may be taken to minimize these risks. Some side effects are hard to prevent, such as the sensation of tingling and/or numbness in the tips of the fingers and toes, called peripheral neuropathy. Culprit drugs include bortezomib (Velcade), cisplatin (Platinol), docetaxel (Taxotere), oxaliplatin (Eloxatin), paclitaxel (Taxol), vinblastine (Velban), and vincristine (Oncovin). Although the symptoms of peripheral neuropathy diminish over time, they may persist, even faintly, for months or years after treatment. Because of this, patients are monitored closely for early symptoms so that the treatment regimen can be altered (if possible) to prevent severe neuropathy. Oncologists may also prescribe medications to alleviate the symptoms, such as amitriptyline (Elavil), nortriptyline (Pamelor), gabapentin (Neurontin), pregabalin (Lyrica), and duloxitene (Cymbalta). The usefulness of supplemental vitamins E, B6, and B12 is under study. Caution: alcoholic drinks may worsen peripheral neuropathy.

Some chemotherapy drugs as well as radiation therapy may contribute to (or directly cause) the development of new cancers many years after treatment. Treatment-related cancers are called secondary cancers. This is not a common occurrence, although its frequency is not known with certainty because of the difficulty in distinguishing secondary cancers from new cancers that were destined to arise anyway. As more people are cured of cancer, the true incidence of treatment-related cancers will become clearer. Cancer survivors are routinely monitored for secondary cancers by their health care team (see chapter 8).

If a particular treatment is linked to subsequent cancers, then researchers have tried to find equally effective alternatives. An example would be the change from a chemotherapy regimen called MOPP to another one named ABVD for the treatment of Hodgkin lymphoma; ABVD offers a lower risk of leukemia and even better outcomes. Also, lower doses of radiation are now being used to treat Hodgkin lymphoma in order to minimize the risks of future breast and lung cancers.

Visit www.cancer.net to learn more about the short-term and possible long-term effects of chemotherapy.

Myth: Once chemotherapy is started, it cannot be stopped until the recommended treatment course has been completed.

Fact: As a patient, the decisions to initiate and terminate medical treatments are your own. Chemotherapy may be stopped after the first cycle, the first injection, the first pill. If you are a patient and you feel strongly about terminating treatments prematurely, then it is extremely important that you discuss your reasons for doing so with your oncologist. It may be possible to rectify unpleasant reactions to treatment or change the therapy to a more acceptable alternative. If in the end, you wish no further treatment, the oncologist should honor and respect your wishes. Yet the end of cancer treatment does not mean the end of patient care; ongoing physical symptoms and emotional distress caused by cancer will still need to be addressed. Good communication is the key to a rewarding and strong patient-physician relationship.

In conclusion, chemotherapy saves lives. It can cure some cancers and extend survival in many others. But the drugs can be unpleasant and cause unwanted side effects, even though the "chemotherapy experience" has dramatically improved in recent years. And it has been known for decades that chemotherapy alone cannot eradicate the advanced stages of the most common cancers. For this reason, researchers have been dissecting the molecular details of cancer cells in the hopes of uncovering targets for more selective and, it is hoped, more effective drugs. The targeted therapies that have resulted have already begun to revolutionize the management of cancer.

Targeted Therapies

◆ A seventy-five-year-old woman with non-Hodgkin's lymphoma was experiencing weakness and discomfort from enlarged lymph nodes in her neck. She had numerous other medical problems, and her health was too poor for chemotherapy. She received a targeted therapy called Rituxan for one month. She experienced only mild fatigue from the medicine. Her lymphoma responded completely, and she remains without evidence of the disease six years later.

◆ A sixty-five-year-old man developed a recurrence of kidney cancer twenty years after it was removed. The cancer was extensive in his liver and pancreas, and he was extremely weak; it did not respond to interferon, and chemotherapy was felt to be useless. He was treated with a targeted pill called sunitinib (Sutent). Almost overnight he felt better, and after two months his cancer had shrunk dramatically in size. The cancer was controlled in this way for two years, with minimal side effects from treatment.

♦ A fifty-year-old woman was admitted to our hospital with fever, abdominal pain, and jaundice. Her health had been declining for several months; now she could barely walk and couldn't eat. She was found to have colon cancer that had formed extensive metastases throughout the liver. We initiated treatment with three chemotherapy drugs (known as FOLFOX) plus a targeted therapy called bevacizumab (Avastin). After a week she could leave the hospital. After two months of regular treatments, she was pain-free, gaining needed weight, and back to full activity levels. CT scans showed that the liver tumors had shrunk by more than 50 percent. After six months of treatment the liver tumors were barely detectable.

TARGETING THE CANCER GENERATOR

The best way to cure a medical disorder is to understand its causes and then block or reverse them. For example, coronary artery disease can be caused by too much cholesterol (along with other risk factors); one way to lower cholesterol levels is with "statin" drugs, which block an enzyme critical for its synthesis in the liver. Ulcers are caused, in part, by excess stomach acid; drugs that block the molecules responsible for acid production, such as omeprazole (Prilosec), help heal ulcers. The targeted therapy of many human ailments has proven to be effective and safe. A similar approach to the treatment of cancer has been the light at the end of the tunnel of cancer researchers for the past fifty years.

Cancer is caused by the misfiring of genes, as discussed in chapter 4. Some genes are overactive, leading to excessive cell growth, whereas others are underactive, allowing this growth to be unrestrained. Thus most targeted cancer therapies aim to shut down the function of an overactive gene or replace an underactive one (this is much more difficult).

Many of the overactive genes are part of the communications network I described above; they give rise to receptors and signaling molecules that are always turned on. Like an electrical circuit that cannot be shut off, overactive receptors and signaling molecules repetitively fire, creating supercharged cancer cells that have their own internal generators. The drugs described below aim to stop these misfirings: the result may be the restoration of calm and the slowing of growth or, better yet, the death of cancer cells. There are thousands of potential targets in cancer cells; advances in chemistry and computing are greatly accelerating the discovery of drugs that can bind to many of them. This class of drugs will likely represent the great bulk of new cancer therapies in coming years.

TARGETING RECEPTORS

Drugs like cetuximab (Erbitux) for colorectal and head and neck cancers, rituximab (Rituxan) for lymphoma, and trastuzumab (Herceptin) for breast cancer are administered intravenously. Once in the bloodstream, they act like heat-seeking missiles, locating cancer cells wherever they lurk and gripping onto them via one specific receptor target (among thousands of receptors) that projects from the outer surface of the cells. The result is that the receptors stop transmitting growth signals inside cancer cells.

Many drugs in this class are modifications of large molecules called antibodies, which our bodies normally generate against infectious agents such as bacteria. Cancer-fighting antibodies are also called monoclonal antibodies. Because of their structural similarity to infection-fighting molecules, cancer-fighting antibodies are also believed to stimulate the immune system to attack cancer cells once they attach to them. Monoclonal antibodies coat the surface of cancer cells, shut down receptor activity, and (hopefully) lead to cancer cell death (fig. 15).

A second way to target cancer receptors is with drugs that pass inside the cell and bind to the parts of receptors in direct communication with the inner world of cells. Although the receptor can still receive signals from the outside, it cannot transmit these signals internally if it is

177

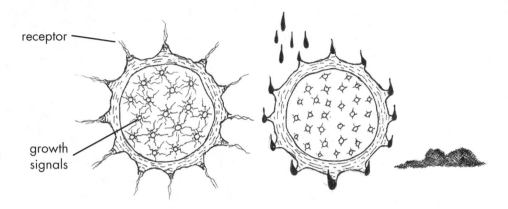

receptor

growth
signals

Fig. 15. *Antibody therapy attacking cancer*
The receptors of a cancer cell (left) are being attacked from the outside by
an antibody therapy (middle), resulting in cell death (right). Illustration
© Gale V. Parsons.

bound by these drugs. The drugs in this class are commonly called small
molecule inhibitors because they can pass freely into cells (their small
size also allows them to be given as pills). Examples include erlotinib
(Tarceva), approved for lung and pancreatic cancer; sunitinib (Sutent),
approved for kidney cancer and GIST tumors; and lapatinib (Tykerb),
approved to treat breast cancer (fig. 16).

TARGETING SIGNALING MOLECULES

The communications pathway from surface receptors to DNA involves
hundreds of different molecules. Silencing a critical signaling molecule
in this network can disrupt the growth and survival signals on which
cancer cells rely. Without these signals, cancer cells can die.

By analogy, suppose a courier has to deliver a package on the other
side of a river and has to cross a bridge. But when he arrives at the
bridge, he finds that it has collapsed; the package will not reach its destination. By shutting down important targets that a growth signal must
use to travel inside a cell, drugs called signal transduction inhibitors
effectively "collapse bridges" throughout cancer cells (fig. 17). Examples

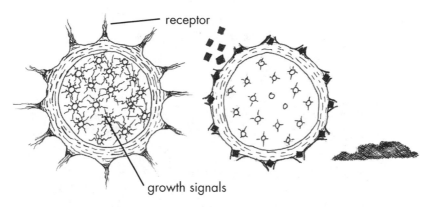

Fig. 16. *Small molecule drugs attacking cancer*
The receptors of a cancer cell (left) are being attacked from the inside of the cell by a small molecule drug (middle), which causes the death of the cell (right). Illustration © Gale V. Parsons.

of signal transduction inhibitors include imatinib (Gleevec) for CML and GIST tumors and sorafenib (Nexavar) for kidney and liver cancer. Many new drugs in this class of cancer fighters will become available in the future (fig. 17).

TARGETING BLOOD VESSEL GROWTH: ANGIOGENESIS
INHIBITORS

For a cancer to survive, it needs oxygen and nutrients delivered by an adequate blood supply. A growing cancer stimulates certain cells in nearby blood vessels to make new blood vessels for itself. These are called endothelial cells; the process of making new blood vessels is called angiogenesis.

Angiogenesis inhibitors are drugs that stop endothelial cells from forming new blood vessels. They do this by jamming their communications networks. Just as in cancer cells, endothelial cell growth signals are transmitted through receptors and signaling molecules. Drugs such as bevacizumab (Avastin), sunitinib (Sutent), and sorafenib (Nexavar) affect the function of these molecules, causing blood vessels that feed a cancer to wither and die (fig. 18).

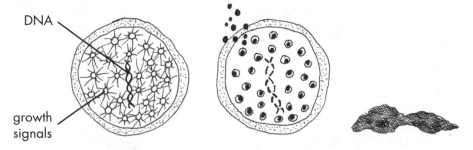

DNA

growth
signals

Fig. 17. *Signal transduction inhibitors attacking cancer*
Growth signals inside a cancer cell (left) are silenced by a class of drugs
called signal transduction inhibitors (middle), leading to cell death (right).
Illustration © Gale V. Parsons.

Angiogenesis inhibitors may also have a *direct* effect against cancer
cells because some of their targets are also present on cancer cells themselves, not just on their surrounding blood supply; they may thus have a
dual cancer-fighting effect.

Q&A: TARGETED THERAPIES

Question: Are targeted therapies "magic bullets"?

Answer: Although targeted therapies were developed with the hope
that they would be magic bullets that would neatly eradicate cancer
through the selective targeting of one critical molecule, in general they
have fallen short of this lofty goal. No cancer is considered curable by
treatment through a targeted therapy alone, except perhaps for some
cases of CML treated with Gleevec. This does not mean that targeted
therapies have not helped many cancer patients, because they have. It
probably means that the bar was set too high and that researchers expected targeted therapies to be "home runs" instead of the singles and
doubles they have turned out to be.

The reason for the muted success of targeted therapies is that most
cancers are caused not by one genetic derangement but by several; no
one target functions as an Achilles heel. The next generation of targeted
therapies is being designed to block several communication molecules

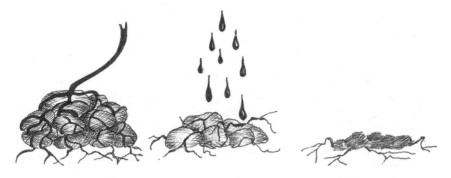

Fig. 18. *Depriving cancer of a blood supply*
A growing cancer is fed by a blood supply (left); angiogenesis inhibitor drugs
deprive cancer of its blood supply (middle), causing the cancer to die (right).
Illustration © Gale V. Parsons.

from functioning. In this way the "magic bullet" concept will likely give
way to the "magic shotgun."

Question: Can targeted therapies be used instead of chemotherapy?

Answer: Targeted therapies have not eliminated the need for chemotherapy. The three patient vignettes presented at the beginning of this
section illustrate the three uses of targeted therapies: (1) as an alternative to chemotherapy when both have activity against a cancer (such as
in low-grade lymphomas, when Rituximab alone may be an effective
therapy); (2) where chemotherapy has a limited role (such as in kidney
cancer and GIST tumors); and (3) to complement chemotherapy (such
as in breast, lung, and colorectal cancers).

> *The combination of the most effective chemotherapy drug(s) plus a*
> *targeted therapy is becoming a prevalent way to treat cancer.*

For example, because all cancers need a blood supply to grow, angiogenesis inhibitors are being successfully combined with chemotherapy
to treat a broad array of cancers. Because not all targeted therapies work
well with all types of chemotherapies, clinical trials are necessary to
establish which combinations work best.

Question: If angiogenesis inhibitor drugs decrease blood flow to a tumor, how can they improve the effectiveness of chemotherapy?

Answer: For any cancer-fighting drug to work, it must have access to the cancer through the bloodstream. It is therefore counterintuitive that angiogenesis inhibitors, which diminish tumor blood flow, should improve the effectiveness of chemotherapy. Here is one possible explanation why it works: Consider a new ball of string, neatly wound around and around into an organized pattern. Next, imagine giving that ball of string to a playful cat and returning an hour later. You would find a disorganized heap of string, with the strands nicked and torn in many places. Now imagine that the string represents blood vessels: the new ball represents the pattern of blood flow in a normal organ, whereas the string damaged by the cat represents the course of blood vessels in a tumor.

Angiogenesis inhibitors actually help reorganize the frantic pattern of tumor blood vessels by repairing the nicks that make them leaky and diverting blood from the most injured ones. As a result, tumor blood vessels become "normalized," and blood distribution actually improves, though it is diminished overall. The result is that chemotherapy has improved access to cancers when given with angiogenesis inhibitors.

Question: Do targeted therapies cause side effects?

Answer: Like any drug taken for any purpose, unintended effects may occur with these medications. *Generally speaking,* targeted therapies are easier to tolerate—less hair loss, smaller declines in blood counts, and less nausea. For example, Rituxan is much gentler than chemotherapy for lymphoma, and Gleevec causes far fewer side effects than interferon or a stem-cell transplant for CML.

Still, substantial side effects may occur with some targeted therapies, and they tend to increase the toxicities of chemotherapy when used in combination. For example, drugs that block a molecule called the epidermal growth factor receptor (EGFR) on the surface of cancer cells, such as Erbitux, Vectibix, and Tarceva (called "EGFR inhibitors"), often cause an acnelike rash on the face and upper body that may be severe; helpful medicines include topical hydrocortisone cream 1 percent or 2.5

percent, clindamycin 1 percent gel, pimecrolimus cream (Elidel), and oral doxycycline or minocycline twice daily. In the case of severe skin reactions, the targeted medicines may need to be stopped temporarily or their dosages reduced to allow the skin to recover.

Interestingly, some rash is a good thing: patients who develop any rash with EGFR inhibitors usually experience better control of their cancer than those who do not. It is important to inform your oncologist when a faint rash begins and not wait until it has become very bothersome and prominent; early intervention is the best way to prevent severe skin reactions.

Another type of skin reaction to cancer-fighting medications, called "hand-foot syndrome," may occur with the targeted therapies Sutent and Nexavar as well as with some chemotherapy drugs, such as Xeloda, Doxil, and 5-FU. In hand-foot syndrome, the hands and feet become dry, reddened, painful, and swollen; there may also be skin breakdown and blisters on the palms and soles. Moisturizers and emollient preparations such as Bag Balm and Udder Cream are often helpful, and your oncology team may recommend other measures. Again, early intervention is the key to preventing severe hand-foot syndrome.

Finally, angiogenesis inhibitors constrict blood vessels not only inside tumors but also in other parts of the body. As a result, they often cause some degree of high blood pressure (which may require antihypertensive medication) and are associated with an increased risk for kidney damage, bleeding, stroke, and coronary artery blockage. Patients with a history of these or other medical conditions may not be suitable candidates for these drugs.

Your oncologist will discuss the possible benefits and risks of taking any targeted therapy with you. As always, the choice of cancer therapy depends on the optimal treatment for the disease, your health, and your preferences.

Visit www.cancer.net and other web sites listed in appendix 2 to learn more about managing the side effects of targeted therapies.

Question: Will targeted therapies be tailored to each patient in the future?

Answer: Patients want to take drugs that will work for them, and doctors only want to prescribe such drugs. The advent of targeted therapies offered the promise of matching the choice of cancer-fighting drug to measurable characteristics of a patient's cancer. For example, if drug A targets molecule Z on cancer cells, then those cancers with the most Z should respond the best to drug A. But in what has been the source of great frustration to patients, physicians, and researchers, this simple relationship has not held up for many targeted therapies.

For example, Erbitux binds specifically to EGFR. Yet the amount of EGFR on a person's cancer cells does not predict how well the cancer will respond to Erbitux. Similarly, Tarceva and Iressa are small molecule inhibitors of EGFR that are used to treat lung cancer; the likelihood of a cancer responding to these drugs is only weakly related to the levels of EGFR present on the cancer cells.

So what does determine the response to a targeted therapy if not the presence of the target? It turns out that for several targets, its *structure or shape* rather than its absolute amount best determines how a cancer will respond to a targeted therapy. For example, if a lung cancer contains an abnormal (mutant) form of EGFR, then there is a much greater chance that Tarceva or Iressa will shrink the cancer; such mutations are found in only 10 percent of all non–small cell lung cancers, often in those who either never smoked or stopped smoking more than twenty-five years before their diagnosis.

New techniques are emerging that will make it easier to detect overactive communications pathways or mutations in specific molecules in the tumor specimen of each patient. In the future, cancer therapies will increasingly tailor the medicines chosen to the specific molecular alterations contained in any given cancer rather than relying only on the type of cancer a person has.

Question: Are there other kinds of targeted therapies besides those discussed?

Answer: You've heard the saying, "Build it and they will come." Well, if a target exists in cancer cells, then scientists will try to target it. Hundreds of targeted therapies are currently being tested. Many will target cancer cells directly, and others will target the immune system, tumor blood vessels, or the normal organs in which metastatic cancers grow (such as the bone and liver). Some will be specific to one cancer type, others broadly active against a large number of different cancers. Access to some of these new treatments can be found at www.clinicaltrials .gov.

> *Whenever possible, support cancer research to help bring new therapies to the clinic.*

Hormone Therapies

Breast and prostate cancers are unique among cancers in that they depend for their survival on the body's hormones. The discovery that manipulating the endocrine system could affect the growth of cancer was made in 1896, when a Scottish surgeon named Sir George Beatson reported that several women with advanced breast cancer experienced dramatic shrinkage of their tumors after he removed their ovaries. By performing this surgery, Beatson had removed the major source of the hormone estrogen from the women's bodies. Although estrogen had not yet been discovered, he knew that the ovaries could powerfully influence breast activity after observing that farmers removed the ovaries of cows after they gave birth, causing them to produce milk indefinitely. Fifty years later, other pioneering surgeons found that castration induced remissions of advanced prostate cancer; in these cases, production of the hormone testosterone was drastically reduced.

Researchers continue to focus on ways of manipulating the endocrine system in order to treat or prevent breast and prostate cancers. Surgery to remove the ovaries or testes remains an important weapon. In addition, an expanding array of drugs has become available. Some provide an alternative way of lowering estrogen or testosterone levels, whereas others prevent the hormones from acting once they reach a cancer.

THE BASIS OF HORMONE THERAPY

All hormone treatments ultimately work by blocking the signals generated inside cancer cells by estrogen or testosterone. Like a plant deprived of sunlight and water, hormone-dependent cancers cannot survive without their hormones. Therefore, the therapies that are commonly called "hormone treatments" are actually antihormone treatments.

How does estrogen initiate each menstrual cycle? How does testosterone induce facial hair? Why do these hormones stimulate breast and prostate cancers to grow? Whichever hormone function we consider, they all boil down to the actions of two pairs of molecules: estrogen plus the estrogen receptor (ER) on the female side and testosterone plus the androgen receptor (AR) on the male side. The ER and AR are collectively called hormone receptors.

> *The attachment of a hormone to its receptor inside a cell is like a baseball landing in a mitt.*

In contrast to the growth receptors described before, hormone receptors exist inside cells, not on their surfaces. Once a hormone enters a cell and finds its receptor, the two go together to attach to DNA. This attachment turns on the DNA and results in the activation of a multitude of genes, accounting for the cell's response to that hormone. For example, breast cells respond to rising levels of estrogen during puberty by maturing; breast cancers that contain the ER (75 percent of them) respond to estrogen by proliferating. Regardless of the type of cell affected, all of these hormonal changes are caused by estrogen binding to the ER.

There are two main approaches to stopping the hormonal stimulation of cancer. The first is to reduce the levels of estrogen or testosterone by halting its production. In breast cancer, leuprolide (Lupron), goserelin (Zoladex), and similar medicines prevent the ovaries from making estrogen by blocking cues from the brain that regulate the ovaries. Anastrazole (Arimidex), exemestane (Aromasin), letrozole (Femara), and other aromatase inhibitors prevent fat and other body tissues from making estrogen. In prostate cancer, Lupron and similar medicines prevent the testicles from manufacturing testosterone by blocking cues from the brain that tell them to do so. Ketoconazole prevents the adrenal glands from making testosterone.

The second approach is to prevent the hormone from attaching to its receptor. The following drugs bind to hormone receptors, blocking estrogen and testosterone from binding to them; as a result, these hormones cannot influence cell behavior. In breast cancer, tamoxifen (Nolvadex) binds to the estrogen receptor and blocks estrogen from binding to it. Fulvestrant (Faslodex) binds to the estrogen receptor and causes the cell to destroy the receptor so that estrogen has no target. In prostate cancer, flutamide (Eulexin), bicalutamide (Casodex), and nilutamide (Nilandron), called antiandrogens, attach to the androgen receptor and prevent testosterone from binding to it. The use of Lupron (or similar drugs) plus an antiandrogen is called "complete androgen blockade": Lupron dramatically lowers (but not to zero) the amount of testosterone in the bloodstream, and the antiandrogen prevents any remaining testosterone from binding to its receptor.

Without the hormonal signals that sustain them, breast and prostate cancer cells wither and die (fig. 19).

Radiation Therapy

Radiation therapy (RT) brings waves of energy particles into contact with cancer cells. It can be delivered by an external beam through a machine called a linear accelerator (the most common form of RT), directly implanted into a cancer in the form of radioactive seeds (called brachytherapy), administered intravenously (such as radioactive iodine given for thyroid cancer), or coupled to monoclonal antibodies (such as Bexxar and Zevalin used to treat lymphoma). RT is also used in other ways.

It is tempting to think of radiation therapy as zapping cancer cells much like a laser in *Star Wars* obliterates an enemy ship. In fact, though,

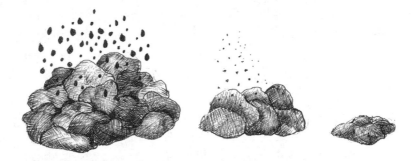

Fig. 19. *Hormone therapy*
Breast and prostate cancers depend on the hormones estrogen and
testosterone to make them grow (left). Hormone therapies decrease the
levels of hormones (middle), resulting in cancer death (right). Illustration
© Gale V. Parsons.

patients receiving RT are told that an MRI or CT scan to assess the
results of their treatment will not be performed for several weeks after
the completion of RT in order to "give the treatment time to exert its
full effect." This is because radiation delivers an energy burst to cells,
setting in motion a number of reactions that over time cause the cell to
die. Just like the drug therapies discussed above, radiation can cause
damage to DNA and interference with the signals communicated inside
cancer cells; it can even exert an angiogenesis inhibitory effect by killing
the endothelial cells that form blood vessels. The result is that RT causes
cancer cells to undergo cell death (fig. 20).

To improve the results with radiation, researchers are studying the
addition of targeted therapies to RT. One of the most impressive results
was recently reported using Erbitux in combination with RT to treat
head and neck cancer. The combination greatly increased survival compared to treatment with radiation alone. The addition of chemotherapy
to this combination is being studied.

Why Do Cancer Treatments Sometimes Fail?

Drug resistance or the growth of cancer in the face of ongoing or recently completed treatments represents the main barrier to cure for

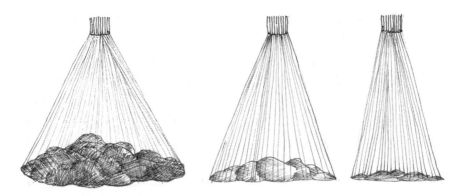

Fig. 20. *Radiation therapy*
Beams of radiation eliminating cancer. Illustration © Gale V. Parsons.

many cancers. When a patient experiences a remission, his or her hopes for cure or prolonged cancer control are naturally raised. It is therefore upsetting and often disorienting to be told that the cancer has relapsed, that the treatments have suddenly stopped working.

In most instances, oncologists cannot specify why a person's cancer develops treatment resistance. We rely on the discoveries of laboratory researchers, who themselves are busy sorting through the myriad of possible scientific reasons for resistance to just one particular drug. If this seems like a bit of double talk, it just might be; treatment resistance is probably the most complicated area of oncology.

The root cause of a cancer relapse lies in the fact that cancer is not an accumulation of exactly the same cells but rather a mixture of cells with differing properties (explained in chapter 5). Some may have sensitivity to certain drugs and be killed by them, whereas others are resistant to those drugs. The resistant population will survive treatment and in time be detected as a cancer relapse. For cancers that can be cured, the available therapies can match all that the cancer can offer by way of resistance. For those that cannot be eradicated, newer treatments are needed that overcome this resistance (see fig. 12).

Drug resistance may be present in an untreated cancer or emerge in response to therapy. In chapter 5, I described the innate adaptability of cancer cells and how they can sometimes outwit an effective therapy by altering their DNA or other molecules. This property explains the acquisition of resistance during a cancer's growth.

Chemotherapy may lose its effectiveness when cancer cells activate a protein that pumps the drugs out as soon as they enter the cells; targeted therapies may lose their ability to control their targets when those receptors and signaling proteins mutate and morph into different shapes; hormone therapies may stop controlling cancer growth when the estrogen or androgen receptors undergo a shape change or get massively overproduced, overwhelming the drugs meant to neutralize them. Through an understanding of the specific genes and proteins responsible for drug resistance, researchers are developing new chemotherapies, targeted therapies, and hormone treatments that may be effective when available treatments stop working.

Exciting new research is shedding light on the "natural" drug resistance of some cancers. Several types of cancer have been found to contain a very small population of cancer stem cells, which are believed to be responsible for continually replenishing the pool of cells in a tumor. It turns out that an additional property of these cancer stem cells is their natural resistance to chemotherapy and other cancer treatments. If the molecules driving the growth of these cells could be specifically targeted by drugs, the treatment of many cancers may improve. The first reported payoff of this approach was presented at the 2008 meeting of the American Association for Cancer Research (www.aacr.org). The study involved patients with aggressive basal cell skin cancer treated with a pill (named GDC-0449) that targets a molecule called "hedgehog." Of the first nine patients enrolled in the study, eight experienced shrinkage or no further growth of their cancer. Targeting cancer stem cells will undoubtedly be an important avenue of research in the years to come.

8

Get Prepared to Survive

At our cancer center we have a ritual to celebrate the completion of each of our patients' cancer treatments. When the last chemotherapy bag has run dry, the oncology nurse escorts him or her to a bell located at the entrance of the infusion suite.

An announcement goes forth: "They're going to ring the bell!" There is a flurry of happy scurrying as staff members rush to join family and friends to witness the momentous occasion. If it's a woman, she may don a diamond tiara (the ninety-nine-cent kind); if it's a man, he'll probably skip that part of the commemoration (or wear it for fun). The patient rings the bell amid a swirl of smiles, cheers, and sincere good feelings.

The release feels great. Perhaps this moment was six months or a year in the waiting. Patients sometimes ring that bell again for emphasis and then hug those whose love and support saw them through; they may shout, raise their arms in victory, cry, or just exclaim, "I'm outta here!"

As the patient leaves the center, however, the familiar path is somehow different. This time the exit leads not just to the outside but to the future—a future that is full of hope but also full of uncertainty.

The transition from the end of treatment to the rest of one's life presents many challenges. Few people can merely "pick up where they left off" the life that they knew before they had to confront cancer. For most, cancer changes everything.

In the past, cancer patients received little guidance about coping in the aftermath of treatment or what to expect from follow-up care. Many survivors felt abandoned once the intensive therapy and check-ups ended. All this is changing. In 2005 the Institute of Medicine, an expert health care advisory panel, issued *From Cancer Patient to Cancer Survivor: Lost in Transition.* This report outlines the many needs of survivors and directions for health care professionals to address them. It recommends that each person completing cancer treatment be counseled and given a treatment plan and summary (called a Survivorship Care Plan) outlining their follow-up care. This plan is to be shared with the patient's primary care doctors to help coordinate care among providers. For patients living with cancer who require ongoing therapy, a modified plan is issued from time to time or when treatment regimens change. The typical care plan contains the following elements:

1. A summary of the patient's diagnosis and treatment history
2. The potential long-term effects from therapy
3. Recommended cancer surveillance (tests and schedules)
4. Healthy living goals
5. Further discussion of family history and need for genetic testing
6. Reassessment of the patient's emotional (psychological) needs and information on the community resources available to address them
7. Reassessment of the patient's practical needs, such as those related to employment and health insurance, and information on resources to address them

I want you to know that the doctors, nurses, social workers, patient advocates, and all those who work with cancer patients understand that almost every patient will face some new psychological, social, and/or physical issue as a result of having to deal with this disease. Many dedicated professionals, volunteers, and organizations are available to assist survivors in dealing with cancer and its many ramifications on their lives. Sadly, many survivors do not find the help they need, either because they don't feel they need it or their physicians do not make the necessary referrals. For example, regarding psychological or emotional counseling, I have heard many patients and family members state, "I wish I had gone for counseling, but I didn't."

It is crucial that all people who are affected by cancer, no matter how strong they may think they are, seek out the appropriate help that will make their long-term recovery as full and vigorous as possible.

Survivorship and the Power of People

From the moment a person is diagnosed with cancer through all of the treatments and then for the rest of his or her life, that person is considered a cancer survivor. The "process" of surviving cancer is called survivorship, and it is indeed a process.

I am not a cancer survivor. Neither am I a counselor or therapist. Yet I have intimately witnessed the effects of this disease on beloved family members and friends. And I have cared for and learned from many people who have fought hard against cancer. Each has his or her own needs and each will handle the ordeal in his or her own way. I and all those who participate in caring for people with cancer are humbled and renewed every day by bearing witness to the tremendous power of the human spirit and the unbelievable generosity of the human heart. I have seen people rise above great adversity, marshal their physical strength and mental toughness, and smile. I have seen women lose beautiful hair (and more of course) and laugh. I have seen vigorous men made weak but still smile and in time regain their vitality. And when the fight against cancer cannot be won, I have seen people die with tremendous dignity, doing it their way, surrounded by love. I have seen their friends and family turn grief into generous acts of volunteering and fund-raising. I have seen people meet these challenges because life is our most precious gift, worth fighting for and worth remembering. As Max Ehrmann wrote in the poem "Desiderata," "With all its sham, drudgery and broken dreams, / it is still a beautiful world." Cancer may challenge us, but it cannot destroy our spirit and who we are. This I have learned.

I have also come to learn of a special force, which I now call "the power of people." Although our religious beliefs may differ, one mystical occurrence that I am certain exists for us all is the power of people. When a volunteer gives a cancer patient a cup of coffee and a smile, when one patient calms the fears of another, when women with cancer get together to put on makeup, when a patient says to me, "I am praying for you and your family," when a boss tells an employee battling cancer, "Take as much time as you need, your job will be here for you," when a nurse makes a home visit to a patient in the middle of the night to alleviate pain, when the local fire department sends a truck and firefighters to celebrate the birthday of a young boy whose mother is battling cancer, when neighbors drop off meals for months on end to a family in need, when entire religious congregations pray for the health of someone they may not even know, when a thousand cancer survivors walk to celebrate life, everyone is lifted up. The power of people: magical, mystical, real. If you have cancer and feel like withdrawing into a shell, you can do that for a time. Then reach out and make the human connections that will help you heal.

PATTERNING YOUR LIFE AS A SURVIVOR

Survival is all about living, how you live day to day despite cancer. In chapter 4, I introduced the term "pattern for living" to describe each individual's daily habits and thought patterns. Once cancer strikes, one's pattern for living is absolutely altered by virtue of having to deal with the psychological and physical impact of the diagnosis. Yet cancer brings to the fore a powerful life force that makes one want to live more than ever. For some, maintaining as much normality as possible is the optimal way to savor life. Others, however, may feel sufficiently shaken by the diagnosis to want to make changes in their lives.

But will these changes be only temporary? What about after the initial period of shock and later acceptance of the diagnosis? What about after treatment ends, or if treatments continue off and on for years? Can the same patterns for living that held sway before cancer continue afterward?

These are the critical questions that each survivor will have to ask him or herself. Certainly, cancer causes fear for one's health and life, for one's very being. But for most people, life will go on after cancer is diagnosed, and so I suggest that each survivor ask him or herself, *"Do I need to make any changes to my life? Can I use cancer as a turning point?"*

Cancer can provide the pause you need to look at how you take care of your body, deal with the stresses of life, and cope with emotional challenges that may have been simmering for years. Did you worry excessively about your life before cancer? Are there personal relationships that need attention and repair? Does your job fulfill you to the extent it should?

When you hear people say things like "Cancer made me a better person" or "Cancer was the best thing that ever happened to me," instead of thinking that these people are half-baked, realize that what they mean is that they used the challenge of cancer to jar their life into a better place. You can, too. Use the positive forces around you along with your own inner strength to change a dysfunctional pattern of living, to make good choices for your life. You will feel better for it and have more peace of mind to cope with cancer as a result.

As a cancer survivor, you will face many challenges. Two of the most important types are physical and psychological (emotional).

PHYSICAL CHALLENGES

The physical challenges facing survivors fall into two main categories: (1) recovery from the side effects of treatment; and (2) monitoring the body for a cancer recurrence or new cancer.

Recovery from treatment. The first aspect of recovery from the physical side effects of cancer treatment involves improving your general health. It is important to recognize that you may need to change your lifestyle.

In the book *After Cancer Treatment: Heal Better, Faster, Stronger,* Dr. Julie Silver, a specialist in rehabilitation and physical medicine at Harvard Medical School and a breast cancer survivor, writes that the three most important physical aspects of a healing lifestyle are:

1. Exercising regularly in a manner that builds strength and endurance
2. Eating a healthy diet
3. Obtaining proper rest during the day (by pacing yourself) and at night (by sleeping well)

Silver advocates making exercise a regular part of your life in order to derive its many benefits: less fatigue, reduction in pain, more strength, improved self-image, enhanced immune function, and decreased risk of developing cancer, among others. Ask your oncologist about resources in your community (such as physical therapy programs and nutrition counseling), and consult the references in appendix 2 so that you can achieve the three essential physical aspects of a healing lifestyle.

The second aspect of physical recovery involves coping with specific problems wrought by cancer treatment. Surgery may have resulted in new physical limitations that may benefit from a consultation with a physiatrist (doctor specializing in rehabilitation medicine) and a program of physical therapy. Cancer-fighting medications and radiation therapy *may* have long-term effects on different body systems, including the health of the heart, bones, brain (cognitive impairment), nerves, and reproductive organs (sexual dysfunction and infertility). You will be informed of these potential side effects both before and especially after treatment, when any preventative measures and a schedule for monitoring these systems (such as a bone density test to assess bone strength) are laid out in your post-treatment care plan. Your primary care physicians and other specialists should also be involved in the post-treatment recovery plan. Several resources listed in appendix 2 discuss in detail the possible long-term side effects of cancer treatment.

Monitoring for recurrences or new cancers. The last thing you want to hear out of the mouth of the oncologist after finishing cancer treatment is, "Well, now it's time for that screening colonoscopy!" Many an on-cologist has received a look in response that basically says, "Go jump in the lake!"

Monitoring for a cancer recurrence and for new cancers that can af-fect all people is an important component of survivorship. Monitoring (also called surveillance) serves two purposes: (1) to try to detect any developing cancer at its earliest stage; and (2) to help alleviate the con-cern over recurrences that all survivors experience. Your survivorship care plan will include both routine cancer screening tests, such as colon-oscopy, mammography, and PSA measurements, as well as specialized tests (such as CT scans and MRIs) to detect a recurrence of the cancer just treated. The guidelines for cancer monitoring often change, so this aspect of your care plan may need to be updated from time to time.

PSYCHOLOGICAL (EMOTIONAL) CHALLENGES

Your psychological state in each stage of survivorship will be different. When initially diagnosed, one must deal with fear and, in some cases, shock and disbelief. At this time, efforts are aimed at developing a treat-ment plan, a plan of action to survive the cancer. During treatment, the focus shifts to surviving the side effects and trying to be positive and hopeful. If treatments continue for a prolonged period, one must adjust one's body and mind, make the cancer center a second home, and cope with the chronic side effects of therapy. If treatment is finite, then on its completion, the cancer survivor will work to resolve side effects or adjust to the "new me"; the focus will turn to regaining one's life and trying to reestablish normality.

Perhaps the most dominant psychological issue facing cancer sur-vivors is the fear of recurrence. Not infrequently, oncologists receive worried phone calls from patients who have completed treatment but who feel a new breast lump, lymph node, or symptom reminiscent of when the cancer began. These fears are normal, and it is our job to pro-vide reassurance (and examinations if needed). Anxiety over a recur-rence can never be fully alleviated, but it can be contained. Some ways to manage it are:

1. Try to live more "in the moment" and not excessively preoccupy your mind with thoughts of what was or what may be (practical preparation for the future is of course important). In an inspiring little book called *The Precious Present,* by Spencer Johnson, MD, we are all reminded to look around and appreciate what life has to offer today, for this is the path to true contentment.

2. Pursue professional counseling with therapists familiar with cancer issues, as discussed below.

3. Counsel another patient who is going through something you may have experienced (peer-to-peer counseling). You may gain a sense of control that is empowering and feel good that you are helping another person through cancer. Peer counselors need to be trained by professionals in order to provide this kind of support to another patient.

4. Gain as much knowledge and understanding of the cancer as possible so that you can focus on the known facts rather than exaggerated fears of recurrence.

5. Use the images in this book to practice guided imagery and focus on the cancer being eradicated or staying away.

6. Separate the anxiety of cancer from anxiety caused by other aspects of your life and seek solutions to those.

The emotional or psychosocial issues generated by cancer are numerous. Distress and anxiety is universal; feelings of isolation and depression are common. How should you best handle these? Sometimes medications may improve symptoms, so you should not hesitate to take prescribed antidepressant or antianxiety medications, which may only be needed for a limited time.

Always the solution involves people. Family, friends, and loved ones sustain us throughout life and especially when we are dealing with cancer. Yet you should also seek out other patients and experienced professionals who are familiar with the emotional toll of cancer. Seeking guidance from oncology-trained psychiatrists, social workers, and psychologists, family therapists, and spiritual or religious advisers will lessen your burdens. It is also beneficial to seek out others who are coping with cancer, because they understand what is happening to you in a unique way. There are many committed and caring people whose job and purpose is to help those with cancer cope from day to day. Yet you must reach out for help or accept assistance when it is offered.

Many cancer patients and their loved ones can benefit from individual or family counseling. Counseling may be limited and used as a bridge until life becomes more normal again or for an extended period. Whether you need simply to talk about your fears or release the stress that may be interfering with a relationship, counseling can start the healing process and avoid letting negative feelings fester and remain unresolved. Oncology counselors are familiar with both the stress created by cancer and the range of family dynamics. Counselors are available at cancer centers as well as through other organizations listed in appendix 2.

One of the best places to find cancer survivors at all stages of the journey is in a cancer support group. You may be reluctant to join such a group. Usually, such reluctance stems from a range of concerns, one of which is a misconception of what a group has to offer. According to oncology social worker Joan Hermann, "Many prospective group members worry that they will hear sad stories and become depressed when what they need is to feel positive and upbeat about their future. While they certainly may hear about the challenges people are experiencing in controlling their cancer, members can also be inspired by the courage and tenacity of others."

Group leaders at our cancer center, Nancy Gennaro, LCSW (licensed clinical social worker), and Michelle Dailey, LMFT (licensed marital and family therapist), liken the experience of joining a group to "the story of the person sitting alone in a boat in the middle of a foggy lake only to discover when the fog lifts, that hundreds of other boaters are all around him." The support group tackles such issues as how to relate to a spouse, child, coworker, or friend; how to summon the energy to work; how to survive when you can't go to work; how to communicate with your doctors; and whom you can count on during these difficult times. The experience is often educational and very rewarding as special bonds are formed.

Survival Is Spelled LMNOP

In this book I convey an understanding of cancer in order to promote an enhanced sense of control over a disease known for the lack of control it creates. I also indicate how diet, exercise, and lifestyle can influence the chances of developing and surviving the disease. The five major elements of preventing and surviving cancer can be easily remembered by thinking, "Survival is spelled 'LMNOP.'"

LMNOP
L   is for *Less* fat in one's diet
M   is for *More* fruits and vegetables
N   is for *No* Smoking
O   is for *Organize* your life
P   is for *Physical* exercise

The effects of diet, smoking, and exercise (L, M, N, and P) on the generation and prevention of cancer are also discussed in chapter 4; the resources listed in appendix 2 provide additional information. The specifics of O are listed below.

O IS FOR ORGANIZE YOUR LIFE

Organize your treatment. Choose caregivers whom you like and trust. Choose a treatment center that fits with your practical needs (such as location) as well as your preferences (for example, a community versus large hospital atmosphere). Get a second opinion when recommended by your primary oncologist or for peace of mind; the more life threatening a cancer, the greater the need to hear more than one opinion. Choose one oncologist to be your most trusted adviser and ally to help you make the best decisions at every juncture of your cancer journey; you should feel that you have good and open communication with this physician.

Pay attention to new advances reported in the media and on reliable web sites and discuss these with your doctors. But don't continually second-guess your treatment plan (or let others do so) or bounce from one specialist to another.

If possible, rely on a small group of about three close friends or family members, at least one of whom will be available to accompany you to each treatment.

Organize your loved ones. On hearing the word "cancer," you will think of yourself and you will think of your loved ones. You will immediately wonder how your spouse or significant other, children, siblings, and parents will handle the news. For the sake of everyone involved, seek the counsel of professionals on how to communicate effectively with your loved ones about your situation. The people in your life may also need the emotional support of a professional counselor at some point. The more united your loved ones are behind you, the stronger you will be throughout your ordeal with cancer.

Address advance health care directives through a living will and a power of attorney document so that your wishes will be respected in the event that you will not be able to direct them (a combination document called Five Wishes is available at www.agingwithdignity.org, but be aware that not all states recognize this document).

Organize your support system. You will need the sturdy support of good friends and loved ones to cope with cancer. Rather than having family and friends give you well-meaning but often overwhelming and distracting advice about what you should and should not do to fight cancer, give them concrete suggestions about how they can show their support. Ask that they help in taking care of household chores, meals, child care, transportation to and from treatment, and anything else you may need to help make your life flow smoothly during and after the grind of cancer therapy. Suggest gift certificates to places that you enjoy (you are entitled!).

Organize your mind. Long-term cancer survivors uniformly state that trying to maintain a positive mental attitude is essential to their survival. But there will be down times, both physical and mental, and it is okay to give into them for limited periods. As my mother used to say to me, "Only a fool is happy all the time." Don't let others badger you to be positive and upbeat around the clock, as this will probably only prevent you from expressing your true feelings, leading to worse depression. So surround yourself with people who truly care about you and know how *you* like to communicate. Reduce stress in your life as much as possible and minimize interactions with negative people so that you can focus on the critical task at hand. Pursue spiritual and religious tranquility. Take advantage of hobbies, music, art, yoga, and other activities and techniques to promote relaxation and peace of mind. Celebrate good results. Laugh as much as possible.

Organize your work. You and your employer will want to know how much time you will need to deal with cancer. You may need to work part-time or perhaps sometimes from home, if that is feasible. If arduous treatments are necessary, consider short-term and long-term disability, and know the pros and cons of these. Do not try to maintain a full work schedule and go through rigorous cancer treatments; you will more than likely end up exhausted, compromising both your work and your treatment.

Organize your finances. First, make sure that your medical insurance will cover the prescribed treatments. Your oncologist's office will be able to verify this. Avoid hospitals that are out of your insurance network unless it is essential that you receive care at such a facility; in these instances, letters from your doctors on the necessity of such treatment usually results in insurance coverage. Second, if you are the breadwinner in your family, make certain that your loved ones will be provided for through clear documentation. Even if you are highly likely to survive your cancer, the diagnosis is a good time to get your financial situation in order.

Organize your time. The ultimate goal is for you to have your life so organized that you can deal with cancer treatment almost on autopilot. This will also enable you to have time for yourself, which is an essential component of the recovery process. Once you have taken control of your life as a cancer patient, you will likely never return to taking each day and the gift of life for granted.

Final Thoughts

In closing, I wish to share with you the inspiring wisdom of two special individuals whose words grace the pages of our cancer center newsletter. Elizabeth April-Fritz survived a diagnosis of breast cancer in 1998, a recurrence in 2000, and a second recurrence in 2004 that requires continuous treatment. She writes, "I have learned to share my experience with other people, those who have been diagnosed with cancer and those who are caregivers. I am encouraged to share my learning, my philosophy, my appreciation for life. Each day an anniversary . . . each day a gift. It is amazing to realize that as I write these words and date this submission that it is in fact the eight-year anniversary to the day that I found the original lump in my breast. Eight years later much stronger and wiser and filled with the promise of living life to the fullest."

And from Patricia Taylor, spouse of a colon cancer survivor:

We all share the need to survive—
To remain alive,
To exist,
To carry on despite hardships,
To persevere.
We want to stay usable—
To cope with what we're dealt
To help each other out,
To retain our humanity,
To make some sense of it.

It may not be anything—
It won't replace the life
Broken by cancer,
Like a plate that fell.
And someone hands it back to you,
Saying, "We may be able to put this
back together."

(Or maybe not.)
And once together, never again the same.

But it is something.
Cracks and everything.

Look—
In the end,
And through it all,
Much of what we have
Is simply each other.

Appendix 1: Types of Cancer Medicine

The medicines listed here are grouped according to how they work to fight cancer. The first column lists medications in alphabetical order by generic name followed by trade name in parentheses. The second column lists the cancers for which the medication is used. The corresponding illustrations in the text are indicated. If a medicine you are taking is not listed, ask your doctor to which group it would belong.

Chemotherapy Drugs That Attack Cancer's DNA (see fig. 13)

azacytidine (Vidaza)	MDS, leukemia
altretamine (Hexalin)	ovarian
bendamustine (Treanda)	lymphoma, CLL
bleomycin (Blenoxane)	lymphoma, testicular
capecitabine (Xeloda)	colorectal, breast, stomach, others
carboplatin (Paraplatin)	ovarian, lung, others
carmustine (BCNU)	brain tumors
chlorambucil (Leukeran)	leukemia, lymphoma, CLL
cisplatin (Platinol)	testicular, bladder, esophagus, others
cyclophophamide (Cytoxan)	breast, lymphoma, others

cytarabine	leukemia, lymphoma
dacarbazine (DTIC)	melanoma, Hodgkin lymphoma
daunorubicin	acute leukemia
decitabine (Dacogen)	MDS, leukemia
doxorubicin (Adriamycin)	sarcoma, breast, lymphoma, others
doxorubicin liposome (Doxil)	ovarian, myeloma, sarcoma, breast
epirubicin (Ellence)	breast, stomach
5-fluorouracil (5-FU)	colorectal, head and neck, others
fludarabine (Fludara)	lymphoma, CLL
gemcitabine (Gemzar)	pancreas, lung, bladder, others
ifosfamide (Ifex)	sarcoma, lymphoma, others
irinotecan (Camptosar, CPT-11)	colorectal, lung, esophagus
lomustine (CCNU)	brain tumors
melphalan (Alkeran)	multiple myeloma
methotrexate (MTX)	head and neck, sarcoma, others
mitomycin-C (Mutamycin)	pancreas, lung, others
mitoxantrone (Novantrone)	prostate, lymphoma, others
oxaliplatin (Eloxatin)	colorectal, stomach, pancreas
pemetrexed (Alimta)	mesothelioma, lung
temozolomide (Temodar)	brain tumors, melanoma
topotecan (Hycamtin)	ovarian, lung
vorinostat (Zolinza)	cutaneous T-cell lymphoma (CTCL)

Chemotherapy Drugs That Attack Cancer's Microtubules (see fig. 14)

docetaxel (Taxotere)	breast, lung, prostate, others
etoposide (VP-16)	lung, lymphoma, others
ixabepilone (Ixempra)	breast
nab-paclitaxel (Abraxane)	breast
paclitaxel (Taxol)	breast, lung, ovarian, others
vinblastine (Velban)	lymphoma, testicular, others
vincristine (Onvovin)	lymphoma, sarcoma, others
vinorelbine (Navelbine)	breast, lung, others

Antibodies That Attack Cancer (see fig. 15)

alemtuzumab (Campath)	chronic lymphocytic leukemia
bevacizumab (Avastin)	colorectal, lung, breast
cetuximab (Erbitux)	colorectal, head, neck
denileukin diftitox (Ontak)	T-cell lymphoma
gemtuzumab ozogamicin (Mylotarg)	acute myeloid leukemia
ibritumomab (Zevalin)	B-cell lymphoma
panitumomab (Vectibix)	colorectal
rituximab (Rituxan)	B-cell lymphoma
tositumomab (Bexxar)	B-cell lymphoma
trastuzumab (Herceptin)	breast

Small Molecules That Attack Cancer (see fig. 16)

erlotinib (Tarceva)	lung, pancreas
gefitinib (Iressa)	lung
lapatinib (Tykerb)	breast
sorafenib (Nexavar)	kidney, liver
sunitinib (Sutent)	kidney, GIST

Signal Transduction Inhibitors That Attack Cancer (see fig. 17)

bortezomib (Velcade)*	myeloma, mantle cell lymphoma
dasatinib (Sprycel)	CML, ALL
imatinib (Gleevec)	CML, ALL, GIST, others
nilotinib (Tasigna)	CML
sorafenib (Nexavar)	kidney, liver
temsirolimus (Torisel)	kidney

Drugs Affecting Cancer's Blood Supply (Angiogenesis Inhibitors; see fig. 18)

bevacizumab (Avastin)	colorectal, lung, breast, kidney
lenalidomide (Revlimid)*	multiple myeloma
sorafenib (Nexavar)	kidney, liver

| sunitinib (Sutent) | kidney, GIST |
| thalidomide (Thalomid)* | multiple myeloma |

Hormone Therapies for Breast Cancer (see fig. 19)

aminoglutethimide (Cytadren)
arimidex (Anastrazole)
exemestane (Aromasin)
fulvestrant (Faslodex)
goserelin (Zoladex)
letrozole (Femara)
megestrol acetate (Megace)
tamoxifen (Nolvadex)

Hormone Therapies for Prostate Cancer (see fig. 19)

bicalutamide (Casodex)
flutamide (Eulexin)
goserelin (Zoladex)
ketoconazole (Nizoral)
leuprolide (Eligard, Lupron, Viadur)
nilutamide (Nilandron)

* also work in other ways

Appendix 2: For More Information

1. The Diagnosis and Treatment of Cancer

- Visit the resource room of your local cancer center to find educational booklets on the specific cancer you are interested in.
- Call the Cancer Information Service at 1-800-4-CANCER and request information (this service is sponsored by the National Cancer Institute).
- Visit the National Cancer Institute's (NCI) web site at www.cancer.gov.
- Go to the American Society of Clinical Oncology's patient-oriented web site at www.cancer.net.
- Visit the Leukemia and Lymphoma Society's web site at www.leukemia-lymphoma.org.
- Go to the American Cancer Society's web site at www.cancer.org.

2. Patient Advocacy and Survivorship Groups

Note: These are composed mainly of cancer survivors and other volunteers who provide information, inspiration, and more.

- Visit the Association of Community Cancer Centers' web site at www.accc-cancer.org and click on "Patient Advocacy Groups" to find the groups most relevant to the cancer you are interested in.

♦ Go to the National Coalition for Cancer Survivorship's web site at www .canceradvocacy.org.

♦ Visit the Lance Armstrong Foundation's web site at www.livestrong.org.

3. Patient and Family Support Services

♦ Inquire at your local cancer center about individual or group therapy and counseling for cancer patients and their loved ones (children, spouses, significant others).

♦ CancerCare at www.cancercare.org provides free counseling, information, and financial assistance to patients.

♦ The Wellness Community at www.thewellnesscommunity.org provides counseling and educational programs across the United States and abroad.

♦ The National Hospice and Palliative Care Organization at www.nhpco.org explains hospice and enables you to find hospice agencies in your region.

♦ The Visiting Nurse Associations of America at www.vnaa.org provides access to nursing and home care agencies.

♦ Go to www.accc-cancer.org and click on "Cancer Care Resources."

♦ Visit the web sites listed under 1 and 2, above.

4. Clinical Trials

Note: Only some of the trials available at any cancer center are listed on the Internet.

♦ Ask your oncologist or the research nurses at your local cancer center about clinical trials at that location.

♦ Go to the web sites of the different cancer centers in your area.

♦ Visit the National Cancer Institute's web site at www.cancer.gov to find information about participating in a clinical trial and to access the largest nonprofit database of trials in the United States.

♦ Go to www.emergingmed.com, which helps match patients to appropriate clinical trials.

◆ Visit the TrialCheck web site at www.CancerTrialsHelp.org for the most up-to-date information on cancer clinical trials.

5. Genetic Testing for Cancer Susceptibility

◆ Inquire at your local cancer center about genetic testing or contact the National Society of Genetics Counselors at www.nsgc.org for a listing of genetics counselors in your area who specialize in cancer.
◆ Go to the interactive government web site www.understandingrisk.cancer .gov to learn about your personal risk factors for developing cancer.
◆ Visit www.facingourrisk.com to determine your risk of breast and ovarian cancers.
◆ Go to www.cancer.net to learn more.

6. Nutrition, Exercise, and Cancer

◆ Visit the American Institute for Cancer Research's web site at www.aicr.com for up-to-date information and resources.
◆ Go to Cancer Nutrition Info at www.cancernutritioninfo.com for sound nutritional advice during and after treatment.
◆ Consult the book *Eating Well, Staying Well during and after Cancer,* by Abby Bloch, PhD, RD, et al. (American Cancer Society, 2003), which contains sound advice without the exaggerated claims of many "nutrition and cancer" books.
◆ Consult the book *After Cancer Treatment: Heal Faster, Better, Stronger,* by Julie K. Silver, MD (Johns Hopkins University Press, 2006).
◆ Visit the web sites listed under 1 and 2, above.

Glossary

acute lymphoblastic leukemia (ALL): The most common cancer in children, in whom it is highly curable with chemotherapy. Adult ALL is less common and requires an allogeneic stem cell transplant to achieve cure.

acute myelogenous leukemia (AML): The most common acute leukemia in adults, mainly affecting those sixty years of age and older. Treatment often involves intensive chemotherapy and a stem cell transplant to achieve cure.

adjuvant therapy: Cancer treatments administered after surgery in order to prevent a cancer recurrence.

allogeneic stem cell transplant: The transfer of blood stem cells from one individual (donor) to another (recipient), after treatment of the donor with specific medications; used in the treatment of blood and lymph cancers affecting the bone marrow, such as leukemia.

anemia: Condition when the amount of red blood is lower than the normal range; may contribute to fatigue. Anemia has numerous possible causes, one of which is the administration of chemotherapy.

angiogenesis inhibitors: Cancer-fighting medicines that block the blood supply to a cancer.

apoptosis: The biologic term for the organized process of death experienced by cancer cells in response to cancer-fighting treatments.

autologous stem cell transplant: The removal and return of one's own blood stem cells, separated by the administration of intensive ("high dose") chemotherapy to treat blood and lymph cancers, testicular cancer, and some sarcomas.

blood stem cells: The population of cells derived from bone marrow that can reconstitute a person's bone marrow, blood-forming capacity, and immune system when their own bone marrow has been intentionally destroyed or suppressed as part of the transplant process. Blood stem cells can be driven into the bloodstream and harvested through a catheter in a vein.

bone scan: A radiology test that detects cancer deposits in the bone through the intravenous injection of a radioactive bone-seeking compound.

cancer clinical trial: A research study that enrolls people on a voluntary basis to test the effectiveness of a new way to prevent, diagnose, or treat cancer.

cell: The basic structural building block of all living things.

chromosomes: Rodlike structures found in most living cells that is composed of DNA and proteins required to maintain the DNA. Most human cells have forty-six chromosomes; alterations of normal chromosome structure are commonly found in cancer cells.

chronic lymphocytic leukemia (CLL): The most common type of leukemia, mainly affecting those sixty years of age and older.

chronic myelogenous leukemia (CML): A type of leukemia characterized by an initial chronic phase followed, if not successfully treated, by a more aggressive phase. CML is highly treatable with targeted medicines such as Gleevec.

CT (computerized tomography) scan: Detailed pictures of the inside of the body taken using a sophisticated X-ray machine linked to a computer.

cure: When no evidence of a cancer can be found after treatment for the life of the patient. A cancer is commonly described as cured after a period of time after which the chance of a recurrence is extremely low, such as five or ten years.

EGFR (epidermal growth factor receptor): A molecule on the surface of many cancers that stimulates the cancer to grow; it is the target of a class of cancer-fighting drugs, called "EGFR inhibitors," that include such medicines as Tarceva and Erbitux.

genetic testing for cancer: The analysis of a person's DNA, derived from a simple blood test, to determine their predisposition to develop specific cancers.

The results may enable the person tested and/or his or her family members to prevent cancer if recommended precautions are taken.

genomics: The study of a cancer's DNA through sophisticated scientific techniques.

informed consent: The process by which a person is fully informed and educated about the risks and benefits of a procedure they may undergo; usually relates to participation in a clinical trial or when considering genetic testing for a family cancer gene.

LDH (lactate dehydrogenase): An easily measurable chemical found in the bloodstream that may be generated in high amounts by rapidly growing cancers, in particular lymphomas.

mediastinum: The area of the human body located in the middle of the chest between the lungs, containing the heart, portions of the aorta and vena cava, main bronchial tubes, thymus gland, lymph nodes, and other structures.

metastasis: The spread of cancer to regions of the body away from the original site of the cancer, for example, when colon cancer spreads to the liver.

MGUS (monoclonal gammopathy of undetermined significance): Condition when an M-spike is detected in the bloodstream but there is no evidence of cancer; patients must be followed for the possible development of multiple myeloma and related disorders.

micrometastases: Cancer deposits that have spread in the body but are too small to be detected by imaging techniques, such as CT scans.

M-protein (also called M-spike): An abnormal protein found in the bloodstream of patients with multiple myeloma, Waldenstrom's macroglobulinemia, and some other blood/lymph cancers; the protein is made by the cancerous cells and declines in amount with effective treatment. May also be found in MGUS.

MRI (magnetic resonance imaging) scan: Detailed pictures of the inside of the body taken using a sophisticated machine that uses a powerful magnet linked to a computer.

mutation: A change in the DNA sequence that may alter the function of a gene and its corresponding protein. The DNA of a cancer cell is characterized by the presence of numerous mutations.

neoadjuvant therapy: Cancer treatments administered before and in preparation for surgery.

neutropenia: Condition when the bacteria-fighting blood cells called neutrophils are present in levels significantly below the normal range; usually associated with the use of chemotherapy or radiation. Neutropenia places the patient at increased risk for infection.

oncogenes: Normal genes that function abnormally as a result of genetic mutation and that contribute to the development of cancer; many oncogenes are the targets of new cancer-fighting medicines called targeted therapies.

PET (positron emission tomography) scan: A technique to measure the activity level of some cancers through the injection of radioactive glucose (sugar) into the vein.

primary site: The original location where a cancer begins, for example, the breast, prostate, or lung.

prognostic factor: Some aspect of a patient or their cancer used to predict the aggressiveness and survivability of that cancer; for example, being estrogen receptor (ER) positive is a good prognostic factor in breast cancer.

progressive disease: The term used by doctors to convey that a cancer is growing.

PSA (prostate specific antigen): A blood marker of prostate cancer used in screening for the disease and in following the effectiveness of treatment for metastatic prostate cancer.

radiologist: A physician expert at interpreting imaging test of the human body. A type of radiologist called an *interventional radiologist* is expert at performing procedures (such as the placement of a central venous catheter or the instillation of chemotherapy directly into the liver) under the guidance of an imaging machine, such as a CT scan.

recurrence: Regrowth of a cancer after it has been in remission for some time.

remission: The term used to relate that a cancer has stopped growing and has shrunken in size or amount; in a *partial remission,* the cancer has shrunken by at least 30 percent, whereas in a *complete remission,* no cancer can be detected.

stable disease: When a cancer has stopped growing but has not significantly shrunken in size or decreased in amount.

staging workup: The battery of tests performed to determine the extent of a particular cancer in the body.

stereotactic radiosurgery: A technique in which high-intensity radiation is focused on a small region of the body in order to eradicate a limited area of cancer.

support group: A meeting of cancer survivors or their loved ones, often led by an experienced professional, to help the participants cope with the many effects of cancer on their lives.

survivor: Anyone who has been diagnosed with cancer.

targeted therapy: A type of cancer-fighting medication designed to bind to one or a few critical targets in a cancer cell.

tumor marker: A chemical measured from the bloodstream and made by a particular cancer that is an indirect measure of the growth of that cancer; for example, many testicular cancers generate a marker called AFP.

tumor suppressor genes: Genes that prevent cancer from developing and are commonly inactivated in many cancers. Mutations in tumor suppressor genes are commonly inherited in families with a predisposition to cancer, such as mutations in the BRCA1 and BRCA2 genes in hereditary breast and ovarian cancers.

whole brain radiation therapy: Administration of radiation to the entire brain in order to treat the spread of cancer there.

References

Chapter 1: Understanding Cancer

Alberts, B., et al. *Molecular Biology of the Cell.* 4th ed. New York: Garland Science, 2004.

Armstrong, L., and S. Jenkins. *It's Not about the Bike.* New York: G. P. Putnam's Sons, 2000.

Barr, R. D., and P. J. Fialkow. "Clonal Origin of Chronic Myelocytic Leukemia." *New England Journal of Medicine* 289 (1973): 307–309.

Chambers, A. F., A. C. Groom, and I. C. MacDonald. "Dissemination and Growth of Cancer Cells in Metastatic Sites." *Nature Cancer Reviews* 2 (2002): 563–572.

Cotran, R. S., V. Kumar, and T. Collins. *Pathologic Basis of Disease.* Philadelphia: W. B. Saunders, 1999.

Duvall, E., A. H. Wyllie, and R. G. Morris. Macrophage Recognition of Cells Undergoing Programmed Cell Death (Apoptosis)." *Immunology* 56 (1985): 351–358.

Fialkow, P. J. "The Origin and Development of Human Tumors Studied with Cell Markers." *New England Journal of Medicine* 291 (1974): 26–35.

Fidler, I. J. "Metastasis: Quantitative Analysis of Distribution and Fate of Tumor Emboli Labeled with ¹²⁵I-5-Iodo-2'deoxyuridine." *Journal of the National Cancer Institute* 45 (1970): 773–782.

Fidler, I. J. "The Pathogenesis of Cancer Metastasis: The 'Seed and Soil' Hypothesis Revisited." *Nature Reviews Cancer* 3 (2003): 453–458.

Folkman, J., and R. Kalluri. "Tumor Angiogenesis." In J. F. Holland and E. Frei, eds., *Cancer Medicine,* 161–191. 6th ed. Hamilton, ON: BC Decker, 2004.

Gerlach, M., et al. "Current State of Stem Cell Research for the Treatment of Parkinson's Disease." *Journal of Neurology* 249 (suppl3) (2002): 33–35.

Hahn, W. C., and R. A. Weinberg. "Rules for Making Human Tumor Cells." *New England Journal of Medicine* 347 (2002): 1593–1603.

Hanahan, D., and R. A. Weinberg. "The Hallmarks of Cancer." *Cell* 100 (2000): 57–70.

Holmberg, L., et al. "A Randomized Trial Comparing Radical Prostatectomy with Watchful Waiting in Early Prostate Cancer." *New England Journal of Medicine* 347 (2002): 781–789.

Holmgren, L., M. S. O'Reilly, and J. Folkman. "Dormancy of Micrometastases: Balanced Proliferation and Apoptosis in the Presence of Angiogenesis Suppression." *Nature Medicine* 1 (1995): 149–153.

Janeway, C. A., et al. *Immunobiology: The Immune System in Health and Disease.* New York: Garland, 2001.

Kerr, J. F. R., A. H. Wyllie, and A. R. Currie. "Apoptosis: A Basic Biological Phenomenon with Wide-Ranging Implications in Tissue Kinetics." *British Journal of Cancer* 26 (1972): 239–257.

Li, Y. M., et al. "Upregulation of CXCR4 Is Essential for HER2-Mediated Tumor Metastasis." *Cancer Cell* 6 (2004): 459–469.

Margolis, M., et al. "Racial Differences Pertaining to a Belief about Lung Cancer Surgery." *Annals of Internal Medicine* 139 (2003): 558–563.

Mitka, M. "Is PSA Testing Still Useful?" *Journal of the American Medical Association* 292 (2004): 2326–2327.

Moore, K. L., and T. V. N. Persaud. *The Developing Human: Clinically Oriented Embryology.* 7th ed. Philadelphia: Saunders, 2003.

Norton, L. "Clinical Aspects of Cell and Growth Kinetics." In A. R. Mossa, S. C. Schimpff, and M. C. Robson, eds., *Comprehensive Textbook of Oncology,* 409–414. Baltimore: Williams and Wilkins, 1991.

Nussbaum, R., and C. E. Ellis. "Alzheimer's Disease and Parkinson's Disease." *New England Journal of Medicine* 348 (2003): 1356–1364.

Park, Y. G., et al. "Sipa1 Is a Candidate for Underlying the Metastasis Efficiency Modifier Locus Mtes1." *Nature Genetics* 37 (2005): 1055–1062.

Smith, B. D., et al. "Isolated Needle-Track Recurrence Following Fine Needle Aspiration for Non-Small Cell Lung Cancer." *Journal of Clinical Oncology* 22 (2004): 3828–3829.

Weigelt, B., J. L. Peterse, and L. J. van't Veer. "Breast Cancer Metastasis: Markers and Models." *Nature Reviews Cancer* 5 (2005): 591–602.

Wyllie, A. H., J. F. R. Kerr, and A. R. Currie. "Cell Death: The Significance of Apoptosis." *International Review of Cytology* 68 (1980): 251–306.

Chapter 2: Diagnosis, Staging, Curability

Beer, D. G., et al. "Gene-Expression Profiles Predict Survival of Patients with Lung Adenocarcinoma." *Nature Medicine* 8 (2002): 816–824.

Diamond, J. *Because Cowards Get Cancer Too.* New York: Random House, 1998.

Greene, F. L., et al. *AJCC Cancer Staging Handbook.* 6th ed. New York: Springer-Verlag, 2002.

Jemal, A., et al. "Cancer Statistics." *CA: A Cancer Journal for Clinicians* 55 (2005): 10–30.

Kodish, E., P. A. Singer, and M. Siegler. "Ethical Issues." In V. T. Devita, S. Hellman, and S. A. Rosenberg, eds., *Cancer: Principles and Practice of Oncology,* 2973–2982. 5th ed. Philadelphia: Lippincott-Raven, 1997.

Mayer, R. "Two Steps Forward in the Treatment of Colorectal Cancer." *New England Journal of Medicine* 350 (2004): 2406–2408.

Paik, S., et al. "Gene Expression and Benefit of Chemotherapy in Women with Node-Negative, Estrogen Receptor–Positive Breast Cancer." *Journal of Clinical Oncology* 24 (2006): 3726–3734.

Paik, S., et al. "A Multigene Assay to Predict Recurrence of Tamoxifen-Treated Node-Negative Breast Cancer." *New England Journal of Medicine* 351 (2004): 2817–2826.

Partin, A. W., et al. "Contemporary Update of Prostate Cancer Staging Nomograms (Partin Tables) for the New Millennium." *Urology* 58 (2001): 843–848.

Pennisi, E. "The Ultimate Gene Gizmo: Humanity on a Chip." *Science* 302 (2003): 211.

Ramaswamy, S., et al. "Multiclass Cancer Diagnosis Using Tumor Gene Expression Signatures." *Proceedings National Academy of Sciences USA* 98 (2001): 15149–15154.

Romond, E. G., et al. "Trastuzumab Plus Adjuvant Chemotherapy for Operable HER2-Positive Breast Cancer." *New England Journal of Medicine* 353 (2005): 1673–1684.

Slamon, D. J., et al. "Human Breast Cancer: Correlation of Relapse and Survival with Amplification of the HER2/Neu Oncogene." *Science* 235 (1987): 177–182.

Slamon, D. J., et al. "Use of Chemotherapy plus a Monoclonal Antibody against Her2 for Metastatic Breast Cancer That Overexpresses Her2." *New England Journal of Medicine* 344 (2001): 783–792.

Sledge, G. J., and K. D. Miller. "Exploiting the Hallmarks of Cancer: The Future Conquest of Breast Cancer." *European Journal of Cancer* 39 (2003): 1668–1675.

Williams, M. *The Woman at the Washington Zoo.* New York: Public Affairs, 2005.

Chapter 3: Understanding Specific Cancers

Barille-Nion, S., and R. Bataille. "New Insights in the Biology and Treatment of Myeloma-Induced Bone Disease." In V. Broudy, J. T. Prchal, and G. J. Tricot, eds., *American Society of Hematology Education Program Book,* 255–260. Washington, DC: American Society of Hematology, 2003.

Barlogie, B., et al. "Treatment of Multiple Myeloma." *Blood* 103 (2004): 20–32.

Bartram, C. R. "Chronic Myelogenous Leukemia." In R. Kurzrock and M. Talpaz, eds., *Molecular Biology in Cancer Medicine,* 164–175. London: Martin Dunitz, 1999.

Bradwell, A. *Serum Free Light Chain Analysis.* Birmingham, UK: Binding Site, 2004.

Brennan, M. F., K. M. Alektiar, and R. G. Maki. "Sarcomas of the Soft Tissue and Bone." In V. T. Devita, S. Hellman, and S. A. Rosenberg, eds., *Cancer: Principles and Practice of Oncology,* 1841–1891. 6th ed. Philadelphia: Lippincott Williams and Wilkins, 2001.

Burstein, H. J., et al. "Ductal Carcinoma in Situ of the Breast." *New England Journal of Medicine* 350 (2004): 1430–1441.

Demetri, G. D., et al. "Efficacy and Safety of Imatinib Mesylate in Advanced Gastrointestinal Stromal Tumors." *New England Journal of Medicine* 347 (2002): 472–480.

Druker, B. J., et al. "Efficacy and Safety of a Specific Inhibitor of the BCR-ABL Tyrosine Kinase in Chronic Myeloid Leukemia." *New England Journal of Medicine* 344 (2001): 1031–1037.

Fisher, B., et al. "Tamoxifen in Treatment of Intraductal Breast Cancer: National Surgical Breast and Bowel Project B24 Randomised Controlled Trial." *Lancet* 353 (1999): 1993–2000.

Frank, R. C., and S. D. Nimer. "Transcription Factors and Malignancy." In R. Kurzrock and M. Talpaz, eds., *Molecular Biology in Cancer Medicine,* 147–159. London: Martin Dunitz, 1999.

Frank, R. C., F. Kaplan, and S. Nair. "Response of Carcinoma of Unknown Primary Site Affecting Bone to Thalidomide." *Lancet Oncology* 6 (2005): 534–535.

Greene, F. L., et al. *AJCC Cancer Staging Handbook.* 6th ed. New York: Springer-Verlag, 2002.

Guralnik, D. B. *Webster's New World Dictionary of the American Language.* New York: Simon and Schuster, 1980.

Hegi, M. E., et al. "Mgmt Gene Silencing and Benefit from Temozolomide in Glioblastoma." *New England Journal of Medicine* 352 (2005): 997–1003.

Hodgkin, T. "On Some Morbid Appearances of the Absorbent Glands and Spleen." In A. Holleb and M. B. Randers-Pehrson, eds., *Classics in Oncology,* 21–27. New York: American Cancer Society, 1987.

Jaffe, E. S., et al. *Pathology and Genetics of Tumours of Haematopoietic and Lymphoid Tissues; World Health Organization Classification of Tumours.* Lyon: IARC Press, 2001.

Jemal, A., et al. "Cancer Statistics, 2008." *CA: A Cancer Journal of Clinicians* 58 (2008): 71–96.

Katz, M. H. G., et al. "Tumor-Node-Metastasis Staging of Pancreatic Adenocarcinoma." *CA: A Cancer Journal for Clinicians* 58 (2008): 111–125.

Kyle, R. A., T. M. Therneau, and V. Rajkumar. "A Long-Term Study of Prognosis in Monoclonal Gammopathy of Undertermined Significance." *New England Journal of Medicine* 346 (2002): 564–569.

Lossos, I. S., et al. "Prediction of Survival in Diffuse Large B-Cell Lymphoma Based on the Expression of Six Genes." *New England Journal of Medicine* 350 (2004): 1828–1837.

Miller, V. A., et al. "Bronchioloalveolar Pathologic Subtype and Smoking History Predict Sensitivity to Gefitinib in Advanced Non–Small Cell Lung Cancer." *Journal of Clinical Oncology* 22 (2004): 1103-1109.

Mitelman, F., B. Johansson, and F. Mertens. *Mitelman Database of Chromosome Aberrations in Cancer.* http://cgap.nci.nih.gov/Chromosomes/Mitelman, 2004.

Morrow, M., S. J. Schnitt, and J. R. Harris. "Ductal Carcinoma in Situ and Microinvasive Carcinoma." In J. R. Harris et al., eds., *Diseases of the Breast,* 383-401. Philadelphia: Lippincott Williams and Wilkins, 2000.

Mundy, G. R. "Metastasis to Bone: Causes, Consequences and Therapeutic Opportunities." *Nature Reviews Cancer* 2 (2002): 584-593.

Pavlidis, N., et al. "Diagnostic and Therapeutic Management of Cancer of an Unknown Primary." *European Journal of Cancer* 39 (2003): 1990-2005.

Peggs, K, and S. MacKinnon. "Imatinib Mesylate: The New Gold Standard for Treatment of Chronic Myeloid Leukemia." *New England Journal of Medicine* 348 (2003): 1048-1050.

Plaat, B. E. C., et al. "Soft Tissue Leiomyosarcomas and Malignant Gastrointestinal Stromal Tumors: Differences in Clinical Outcome and Expression of Multidrug Resistance Proteins." *Journal of Clinical Oncology* 18 (2000): 3211-3220.

Raje, N., and K. Anderson. "Thalidomide—a Revival Story." *New England Journal of Medicine* 341 (1999): 1606-1609.

Ramaswamy, S., et al. "Multiclass Cancer Diagnosis Using Tumor Gene Expression Signatures." *Proceedings of the National Academy of Sciences USA* 98 (2001): 15149-15154.

Rassenti, L. Z., et al. "Zap-70 Compared with Immunoglobulin Heavy-Chain Gene Mutation Status as a Predictor of Disease Progression in Chronic Lymphocytic Leukemia." *New England Journal of Medicine* 351 (2004): 893-901.

Sanchez-Beato, M., A. Sanchez-Aguilera, and M. A. Piris. "Cell Cycle Deregulation in B-Cell Lymphoma." *Blood* 101 (2003): 1220-1235.

Shah, N. P., et al. "Overriding Imatinib Resistance with a Novel Abl Kinase Inhibitor." *Science* 305 (2004): 399-401.

Singh, S. K., et al. "Identification of Human Brain Tumour Initiating Cells." *Nature* 432 (2004): 396-401.

Singhal, S., et al. "Antitumor Activity of Thalidomide in Refractory Multiple Myeloma." *New England Journal of Medicine* 341 (1999): 1565-1571.

Sirohi, B., and R. Powles. "Multiple Myeloma." *Lancet* 363 (2004): 875–887.

Tamboli, P., and J. Y. Ro. "Pathologic Evaluation of Lung Cancer." In F. V. Fossella, R. Komaki, and J. B. Puntam, Jr., *M.D. Anderson Cancer Care Series: Lung Cancer,* 57–80. New York: Springer-Verlag, 2003.

Virchow, R. "Cellular Pathology: Blood and Lymph." In A. Holleb and M. B. Randers-Pehrson, eds., *Classics in Oncology,* 55–69. New York: American Cancer Society, 1987.

Visnjic, D., et al. "Hematopoiesis Is Severely Altered in Mice with an Induced Osteoblast Deficiency." *Blood* 103 (2004): 3258–3264.

Williams, P. L., et al. *Gray's Anatomy.* 38th ed. New York: Churchill Livingstone, 1995.

Chapter 4: Why Cancer Develops

Alberts, B., et al. *Molecular Biology of the Cell.* 4th ed. New York: Garland Sciences, 2002.

The Alpha-Tocopherol, Beta Carotene Cancer Prevention Study Group. "The Effect of Vitamin E and Beta Carotene on the Incidence of Lung Cancer and Other Cancers in Male Smokers." *New England Journal of Medicine* 330 (1994): 1029–1035.

Amundadottir, L. T., et al. "Cancer as a Complex Phenotype: Pattern of Cancer Distribution within and beyond the Nuclear Family." *PLoS Medicine* 1 (2004): 229–236.

Bairati, I., et al. "A Randomized Trial of Antioxidant Vitamins to Prevent Second Primary Cancers in Head and Neck Cancer Patients." *Journal of the National Cancer Institute* 97 (2005): 481–488.

Beal, M. F. "Less Stress, Longer Life." *Nature Medicine* 11 (2005): 598–599.

Belani, P. B., and S. Ramalingam. "Smoking Cessation and Treatment Outcome." *Clinical Lung Cancer* (March 2004): 264.

Belitz, H.-D., W. Grosch, and P. Schieberle. *Food Chemistry.* Berlin: Springer, 2004.

Bingham, S., and E. Riboli. "Diet and Cancer: the European Prospective Investigation into Cancer and Nutrition." *Nature Reviews Cancer* 4 (2004): 206–215.

Bishop, J. M. *Nobel Lecture: Retroviruses and Oncogenes II.* http://nobelprize.org/medicine/laureates/1989/bishop-lecture.pdf, 1989: 530–548.

Bloch, A., et al. *Eating Well, Staying Well during and after Cancer.* Atlanta, GA: American Cancer Society, 2004.

Brizer, D. *Quitting Smoking for Dummies.* Hoboken, NJ: Wiley, 2003.

Calle, E. E., and R. Kaaks. "Overweight, Obesity and Cancer: Epidemiological Evidence and Proposed Mechanisms." *Nature Cancer Reviews* 4 (2004): 579–591.

Calle, E. E., et al. "Overweight, Obesity and Mortality from Cancer in Prospectively Studied Cohorts of US Adults." *New England Journal of Medicine* 348 (2003): 1625–1638.

Chakravarti, A., and P. Little. "Nature, Nurture and Human Disease." *Nature* 421 (2003): 412–414.

Chao, A., et al. "Meat Consumption and Risk of Colorectal Cancer." *Journal of the American Medical Association* 293 (2005): 172–182.

Chapelle, A. de la. "Genetic Predisposition to Colorectal Cancer." *Nature Reviews Cancer* 4 (2004): 769–780.

Chlebowski, R. T., et al. "Dietary Fat Reduction and Breast Cancer Outcome: Interim Efficacy Results from the Women's Intervention Nutrition Study." *Journal of the National Cancer Institute* 98 (2006): 1767–1776.

Cole, B. F., et al. "Folic Acid for the Prevention of Colorectal Adenomas: A Randomized Clinical Trial." *Journal of the American Medical Association* 297 (2007): 2351–2359.

Cooney, K. A., and S. B. Gruber. "Hyperglycemia, Obesity and Cancer Risks on the Horizon." *Journal of the American Medical Association* 293 (2005): 233–234.

Czene, K., P. Lichtenstein, and K. Hemminki. "Environmental and Heritable Causes of Cancer among 9.6 Million Individuals in the Swedish Family-Cancer Database." *International Journal of Cancer* 99 (2002): 260–266.

Doll, R., and R. Peto. "The Causes of Cancer: Quantitative Estimates of Avoidable Risks of Cancer in the United States Today." *Journal of the National Cancer Institute* 66 (1981): 1191–1308.

Doll, R., et al. "Mortality in Relation to Smoking: Fifty Years' Observations on Male British Doctors." *British Medical Journal* 328 (2004): 1519–1533.

Ewart-Toland, A., et al. "Identification of Stk6/STK15 as a Candidate Low-Penetrance Tumor-Susceptibility Gene in Mouse and Human." *Nature Genetics* 34 (2003): 403–412.

Friend, S. H., et al. "A Human DNA Segment with Properties of the Gene

That Predisposes to Retinoblastoma and Osteosarcoma." *Nature* 323 (1986): 643–646.

Garber, J. E., and K. Offit. "Hereditary Cancer Predisposition Syndromes." *Journal of Clinical Oncology* 23 (2005): 276–292.

Gils, C. van, et al. "Consumption of Vegetables and Fruits and Risk of Breast Cancer." *Journal of the American Medical Association* 293 (2005): 183–193.

Goldgar, D. E., et al. "Systematic Population-Based Assessment of Cancer Risk in First-Degree Relatives of Cancer Probands." *Journal of the National Cancer Institute* 86 (1994): 1600–1608.

Goodsell, D. S. "The Molecular Perspective: Polycyclic Aromatic Hydrocarbons." *Oncologist* 9 (2004): 469–470.

Gotay, C. G. "Behavior and Cancer Prevention." *Journal of Clinical Oncology* 23 (2004): 301–310.

Greaves, M. "Cancer Causation: The Darwinian Downside of Past Success?" *Lancet Oncology* 3 (2002): 244–251.

Griffiths, K., et al. *Nutrition and Cancer.* Oxford: Isis Medical Media, 1996.

Hahn, W., and R. Weinberg. "Rules for Making Human Tumor Cells." *New England Journal of Medicine* 347 (2002): 1593–1603.

Hanahan, D., and R. A. Weinberg. "The Hallmarks of Cancer." *Cell* 100 (2000): 57–70.

Hauser, S. L., and D. E. Goodkin. "Multiple Sclerosis and Other Demyelinating Diseases." In A. S. Fauci et al., eds., *Harrison's Principles of Internal Medicine,* 2409–2419. 14th ed. New York: McGraw-Hill, 1998.

Heber, D., G. L. Blackburn, and V. L. W. Go. *Nutritional Oncology.* San Diego: Academic, 1999.

Holick, M. F. "Vitamin D Deficiency." *New England Journal of Medicine* 357 (2007): 266–281.

Holmes, M. D., et al. "Physical Activity and Survival after Breast Cancer Diagnosis." *Journal of the American Medical Association* 293 (2005): 2479–2486.

The HOPE and HOPE-Too Trial Investigators. "Effects of Long-Term Vitamin E Supplementation on Cardiovascular Events and Cancer: A Randomized Controlled Trial." *Journal of the American Medical Association* 293 (2005): 1338–1347.

Huhmann, M. B., and R. S. Cunningham. "Importance of Nutritional Screening in Treatment of Cancer-Related Weight Loss." *Lancet Oncology* 6 (2005): 334–343.

Hung, H. C., et al. "Fruit and Vegetable Intake and Risk of Major Chronic Disease." *Journal of the National Cancer Institute* 96 (2004): 1577–1584.

International Human Genome Sequencing Consortium. "Finishing the Euchromatic Sequence of the Human Genome." *Nature* 431 (2004): 931–945.

Jonsson, S., et al. "Familial Risk of Lung Carcinoma in the Icelandic Population." *Journal of the American Medical Association* 292 (2004): 2977–2983.

Judson, H. F. *The Eighth Day of Creation.* Plainview, NY: Cold Spring Harbor Laboratory Press, 1996.

Kaiser, J. "Tying Genetics to the Risk of Environmental Diseases." *Science* 300 (2003): 563.

Kastan, M. B., and J. Bartek. "Cell-Cycle Checkpoints and Cancer." *Nature* 432 (2004): 316–323.

Kemp, M. "The Mona Lisa of Modern Science." *Nature* 421 (2003): 416–420.

Kinzler, K. W., and B. Vogelstein. "Lessons from Hereditary Colorectal Cancer." *Cell* 87 (1996): 159–170.

Klein, E. A., et al. "Select: The Next Prostate Cancer Prevention Trial." *Journal of Urology* 166 (2001): 1311–1315.

Kolata, G. "The Body Heretic: It Scorns Our Efforts." *New York Times,* April 17, 2005, 1–3.

Kroenke, C. K., et al. "Weight, Weight Gain, and Survival after Breast Cancer Diagnosis." *Journal of Clinical Oncology* 23 (2005): 1370–1378.

Lichtenstein, A. H., and R. M. Russell. "Essential Nutrients: Food or Supplements?" *Journal of the American Medical Association* 294 (2005): 351–358.

Lucia, M. S., et al. "Pathologic Characteristics of Cancer Detected in the Prostate Cancer Prevention Trial: Implications for Prostate Cancer Detection and Chemoprevention." *Cancer Prevention Research* 1 (2008): 167–173.

Lynch, H. T., et al. "Hereditary Breast-Ovarian Cancer at the Bedside: Role of the Medical Oncologist." *Journal of Clinical Oncology* 21 (2003): 740–753.

Meyerhardt, J. A., et al. "Impact of Physical Activity on Cancer Recurrence and Survival in Patients with Stage III Colon Cancer: Findings from CALGB 89803." *Journal of Clinical Oncology* 24 (2006): 3535–3541.

Miki, Y., et al. "A Strong Candidate for the Breast and Ovarian Cancer Susceptibility Gene BRCA1." *Science* 266 (1994): 66–71.

National Center for Biotechnology Information. A Science Primer. www.ncbi.nlm.nih.gov/About/primer/snps.html.

Nelson, W., A. M. DeMarzo, and W. B. Isaacs. "Prostate Cancer." *New England Journal of Medicine* 349 (2003): 366–381.

Nussbaum, R. L., R. R. McInnes, and H. F. Willard. *Thompson and Thompson Genetics in Medicine.* 6th ed. Philadelphia: W. B. Saunders, 2001.

Offit, K., et al. *ASCO Curriculum: Cancer Genetics and Cancer Predisposition Testing.* 2nd ed. Alexandria, VA: American Society of Clinical Oncology, 2004.

Rajagopalan, H., and C. Lengauer. "Aneuploidy and Cancer." *Nature* 432 (2004): 338–341.

Ravasco, P., et al. "Dietary Counseling Improves Patient Outcomes: A Prospective, Randomized, Controlled Trial in Colorectal Cancer Patients Undergoing Radiotherapy." *Journal of Clinical Oncology* 23 (2005): 1431–1438.

Redman, M. W., et al. "Finasteride Does Not Increase the Risk of High-Grade Prostate Cancer: A Bias-Adjusted Modeling Approach." *Cancer Prevention Research* 1 (2008): 174–181.

Renan, M. J. "How Many Mutations Are Required for Tumorigenesis? Implications from Human Cancer Data." *Molecular Carcinogenesis* 7 (1993): 139–146.

Schuller, H. M. "Mechanisms of Smoking-Related Lung and Pancreatic Adenocarcinoma Development." *Nature Reviews Cancer* 2 (2002): 455–463.

Skinner, A. M., and M. S. Turker. "Oxidative Mutagenesis, Mismatch Repair and Aging." http://sageke.sciencemag.org/cgi/content/full/2005/9/re3, 2005.

Stucker, I., A. Hirvonen, and I. de Waziers. "Genetic Polymorphisms of Glutathione S-Transferasese as Modulators of Lung Cancer Susceptibility." *Carcinogenesis* 23 (2002): 1475–1481.

Thorgeirsson, T. E., et al. "A Variant Associated with Nicotine Dependence, Lung Cancer and Peripheral Arterial Disease." *Nature* 452 (2008): 638–641.

Ulrich, C. M., and J. D. Potter. "Folate and Cancer-Timing Is Everything." *Journal of the American Medical Association* 297 (2007): 2408–2409.

US Department of Health and Human Services. Office of the Surgeon General. www.surgeongeneral.gov.

Varmus, H. *Nobel Lecture: Retroviruses and Oncogenes I.* http://nobelprize.org/medicine/laureates/1989/varmus-lecture.pdf, 1989: 504–522.

Venkitaraman, A. R. "A Growing Network of Cancer Susceptibility Genes." *New England Journal of Medicine* 348 (2003): 1917–1919.

Vogelstein, B., and K. W. Kinzler. "Cancer Genes and the Pathways They Control." *Nature Medicine* 10 (2004): 789–799.

Vogelstein, B., and K. W. Kinzler. *The Genetic Basis of Human Cancer.* 2nd ed. New York: McGraw-Hill, 2002.

Vogelstein, B., et al. "Genetic Alterations during Colorectal-Tumor Development." *New England Journal of Medicine* 319 (1988): 525–532.

Watson, J. D., and F. H. C. Crick. "A Structure for Deoxyribose Nucleic Acid." *Nature* 171 (1953): 737–738.

Willett, W. C. "Diet and Cancer: An Evolving Picture." *Journal of the American Medical Association* 293 (2005): 233–234.

Willett, W. C. *Eat, Drink, and Be Healthy.* New York: Free Press, 2001.

Willett, W. C. *Nutritional Epidemiology.* New York: Oxford University Press, 1998.

Yoshida, K., and Y. Miki. "Role of BRCA1 and BRCA2 as Regulators of DNA Repair, Transcription, and Cell Cycle in Response to DNA Damage." *Cancer Science* 95 (2004): 866–871.

Zhou, B. S., and S. J. Elledge. "The DNA Damage Response: Putting Checkpoints in Perspective." *Nature* 408 (2000): 433–439.

Zhou, W., et al. "Circulating 25-Hydroxyvitamin D Levels Predict Survival in Early-Stage Non–Small Cell Lung Cancer Patients." *Journal of Clinical Oncology* 25 (2007): 479–485.

Chapter 5: How Cancer Grows

Abraham, S. C., L. J. Burgart, and R. D. Odze. "Polyps of the Large Intestine." In R. D. Odze, J. R. Goldblum, and J. M. Crawford, eds., *Surgical Pathology of the GI Tract, Liver, Biliary Tract, and Pancreas,* 327–329. Philadelphia: Elsevier, 2004.

Allen, J. I. "Colorectal Cancer." In R. Kurzrock and M. Talpaz, eds., *Molecular Biology in Cancer Medicine,* 317–331. London: Martin Dunitz, 1999.

Auerbach, O., et al. "Changes in Bronchial Epithelium in Relation to Cigarette Smoking and in Relation to Lung Cancer." *New England Journal of Medicine* 265 (1961): 253–267.

Dean, M., T. Fojo, and S. Bates. "Tumour Stem Cells and Drug Resistance." *Nature Reviews Cancer* 5 (2005): 275–284.

Fearon, E. R., and B. Vogelstein. "A Genetic Model for Colorectal Tumorigenesis." *Cell* 61 (1990): 759–767.

Greaves, M. "Cancer Causation: The Darwinian Downside of Past Success?" *Lancet Oncology* 3 (2002): 244–251.

Hellman, S., and J. R. Harris. "Natural History of Breast Cancer." In J. R. Harris et al., eds., *Diseases of the Breast,* 407–424. 2nd ed. Philadelphia: Lippincott Williams and Wilkins, 2000.

Morson, B. C. "Polyps and Cancer of the Large Bowel." *Monographs in Pathology* 18 (1977): 101–108.

Mulshine, J. L., and D. C. Sullivan. "Lung Cancer Screening." *New England Journal of Medicine* 352 (2005): 2714–2720.

Nowell, P. C. "The Clonal Evolution of Tumor Cell Populations." *Science* 194 (1976): 23–28.

Vogelstein, B., and K. W. Kinzler. "The Multistep Nature of Cancer." *Trends In Genetics* 9 (1993): 138–141.

Vogelstein, B., et al. "Genetic Alterations during Colorectal-Tumor Development." *New England Journal of Medicine* 319 (1988): 525–532.

Welch, H. G. *Should I Be Tested for Cancer?* Berkeley: University of California Press, 2004.

Welch, H. G., S. Woloshin, and L. M. Schwartz. "Skin Biopsy Rates and Incidence of Melanoma: Population Based Ecological Study." *British Medical Journal* 331 (2005): 481.

Winawer, S., et al. "Prevention of Colorectal Cancer by Colonoscopic Polypectomy: The National Polyp Study Workgroup." *New England Journal of Medicine* 329 (1993): 1977–1981.

Chapter 6: Cancer Treatments Revolve around Metastasis

Allegra, C., and D. Sargent. "Adjuvant Therapy for Colon Cancer: The Pace Quickens." *New England Journal of Medicine* 352 (2005): 2746–2748.

Battaile, J. "Very Much Alive, Thank You." *New York Times,* July 17, 2005, 3.

Bolla, M., et al. "Long-Term Results with Immediate Androgen Suppression and External Irradiation in Patients with Locally Advanced Prostate Cancer (an EORTC Study): A Phase III Randomized Trial." *Lancet* 360 (2002): 103–106.

Burstein, H. J., et al. "Clinical Activity of Trastuzumab and Vinorelbine in Women with Her2-Overexpressing Metastatic Breast Cancer." *Journal of Clinical Oncology* 19 (2001): 2722–2730.

Fisher, B., et al. "Effect of Preoperative Chemotherapy on the Outcome of Women with Operable Breast Cancer." *Journal of Clinical Oncology* 16 (1998): 2672–2685.

Fisher, B., et al. "L-Phenylalanine Mustard (L-PAM) in the Management of Primary Breast Cancer: A Report of Early Findings." *New England Journal of Medicine* 292 (1975): 117–122.

Flanigan, R., et al. "Nephrectomy Followed by Interferon Alfa-2b Compared with Interferon Alfa-2b Alone for Metastatic Renal-Cell Cancer." *New England Journal of Medicine* 345 (2001): 1655–1659.

Goldberg, R. M., et al. "A Randomized Controlled Trial of Fluorouracil Plus Leucovorin, Irinotecan, and Oxaliplatin Combinations in Patients with Previously Untreated Metastatic Colorectal Cancer." *Journal of Clinical Oncology* 22 (2004): 23–30.

Gosney, M. A. "Clinical Assessment of Elderly People with Cancer." *Lancet Oncology* 6 (2005): 790–797.

Green, M., and G. N. Hortobagyi. "Neoadjuvant Chemotherapy for Operable Breast Cancer." *Oncology* (Huntington) 16 (2002): 871–884.

Greenberg, P. A. C., et al. "Long-Term Follow-Up of Patients with Complete Remission Following Combination Chemotherapy for Metastatic Breast Cancer." *Journal of Clinical Oncology* 14 (1996): 2197–2205.

Hellman, S. "Natural History of Small Breast Cancers." *Journal of Clinical Oncology; Classic Papers and Current Comments* 5 (2001): 865–871.

Kamen, B. A., E. Rubin, and J. Aisner. "High-Time Chemotherapy or High Time for Low Dose." *Journal of Clinical Oncology* 18 (2000): 2935–2937.

Motzer, R. J., et al. "Activity of SU11248, a Multitargeted Inhibitor of Vascular Endothelial Growth Factor Receptor and Platelet-Derived Growth Factor Receptor, in Patients with Metastatic Renal Cell Carcinoma." *Journal of Clinical Oncology* 24 (2006): 16–23.

O'Reilly, M. S., et al. "Angiostatin: A Novel Angiogenesis Inhibitor That Mediates the Suppression of Metastases by a Lewis Lung Carcinoma." *Cell* 79 (1994): 315–328.

Ozols, R. F., et al. "Epithelial Ovarian Cancer." In W. J. Hoskins, C. A. Perez, and R. C. Young, eds., *Principles and Practice of Gynecologic Oncology,* 981–1057. 3rd ed. Philadelphia: Lippincott Williams and Wilkins, 2000.

Piccart-Gebhart, M. J., et al. "Trastuzumab after Adjuvant Chemotherapy in HER2-Positive Breast Cancer." *New England Journal of Medicine* 353 (2005): 1659–1672.

Pisters, K. M. W. "Adjuvant Chemotherapy for Non–Small Cell Lung Cancer: The Smoke Clears." *New England Journal of Medicine* 352 (2005): 2640–2642.

Rini, B., et al. "Ag-013736, a Multi-Target Tyrosine Kinase Receptor Inhibitor, Demonstrates Anti-Tumor Activity in a Phase 2 Study of Cytokine-Refractory, Metastatic Renal Cell Cancer (RCC)." *Journal of Clinical Oncology* 23 (suppl) (2005): 380s (abstract 4509).

Romond, E. G., et al. "Trastuzumab plus Adjuvant Chemotherapy for Operable HER2-Positive Breast Cancer." *New England Journal of Medicine* 353 (2005): 1673–1684.

Schrag, D., et al. "An Increasingly Common Challenge: Management of the Complete Responder with Multi-Focal Metastatic Colorectal Cancer." *Journal of Clinical Oncology* 23 (2005): 1799–1802.

Slamon, D. J., et al. "Use of Chemotherapy plus a Monoclonal Antibody against Her2 for Metastatic Breast Cancer That Overexpresses Her2." *New England Journal of Medicine* 344 (2001): 783–792.

Stadtmauer, E. A., A. O'Neill, and L. J. Goldstein. "Conventional-Dose Chemotherapy Compared with High-Dose Chemotherapy plus Autologous Hematopoietic Stem-Cell Transplantation for Metastatic Breast Cancer." *New England Journal of Medicine* 342 (2000): 1069–1076.

Vijver, M. van de. "Gene-Expression Profiling and the Future of Adjuvant Therapy." *Oncologist* 10 (suppl) (2005): 30–34.

Wasil, T., and S. M. Lichtman. "Treatment of Elderly Cancer Patients with Chemotherapy." *Cancer Investigation* 23 (2005): 537–547.

Winton, T., et al. "Vinorelbine plus Cisplatin vs. Observation in Resected Non–Small Cell Lung Cancer." *New England Journal of Medicine* 352 (2005): 2589–2597.

Chapter 7: Cancer Treatments at Work

Allan, J. M. "Mechanisms of Therapy-Related Carcinogenesis." *Nature Reviews Cancer* 5 (2005): 943–955.

Beatson, G. T. "On the Treatment of Inoperable Cases of Carcinoma of the Mamma: Suggestions for a New Method of Treatment, with Illustrative Cases." *Lancet* 2 (1896): 104–107.

Bonner, J. A., et al. "Radiotherapy plus Cetuximab for Squamous-Cell Carcinoma of the Head and Neck." *New England Journal of Medicine* 354 (2006): 567–578.

Carmeliet, P. "Angiogenesis in Life, Disease and Medicine." *Nature* 438 (2005): 932–936.

Dean, M., T. Fojo, and S. Bates. "Tumour Stem Cells and Drug Resistance." *Nature Reviews Cancer* 5 (2005): 275-284.

Devita, V. T., and P. S. Schein. "The Use of Drugs in Combination for the Treatment of Cancer." *New England Journal of Medicine* 1973 (288): 998-1006.

Frantz, R. "Playing Dirty." *Science* 437 (2005): 942-943.

Huntly, B. J. P., and D. G. Gilliland. "Leukaemia Stem Cells and the Evolution of Cancer-Stem-Cell Research." *Nature Reviews Cancer* 5 (2005): 311-321.

Jain, R. K. "Normalizing Tumor Vasculature with Anti-Angiogenic Therapy: A New Paradigm for Combination Therapy." *Nature Medicine* 7 (2001): 987-989.

Kerbel, R. S., and B. A. Kamen. "The Anti-Angiogenic Basis of Metronomic Chemotherapy." *Nature Reviews Cancer* 4 (2004): 423-436.

Lynch, T. J., et al. "Activating Mutations in the Epidermal Growth Factor Receptor Underlying Responsiveness of Non-Small Cell Lung Cancer to Gefitinib." *New England Journal of Medicine* 350 (2004): 2129-2139.

Lynch, T. J., et al. "Epidermal Growth Factor Receptor Inhibitor-Associated Cutaneous Toxicities: An Evolving Paradigm in Clinical Management." *Oncologist* 12 (2007): 610-621.

Perez-Soler, R., and L. Saltz. "Cutaneous Adverse Effects with HER1/EGFR-Targeted Agents: Is There a Silver Lining?" *Journal of Clinical Oncology* 23 (2005): 5235-5246.

Pham, D., et al. "Use of Cigarette-Smoking History to Estimate the Likelihood of Mutations in Epidermal Growth Factor Receptor Gene Exons 19 and 21 in Lung Adenocarcinomas." *Journal of Clinical Oncology* 11 (2006): 1700-1704.

Polyak, K., and W. C. Hahn. "Roots and Stems: Stem Cells in Cancer." *Nature Medicine* 12 (2006): 296-300.

Prise, K. M., et al. "New Insights on Cell Death from Radiation Exposure." *Lancet Oncology* 6 (2005): 520-528.

Solit, D. B., et al. "BRAF Mutation Predicts Sensitivity to MEK Inhibition." *Science* 439 (2006): 358-362.

Stockwell, S. "Sir George Thomas Beatson, MD (1848-1933)." In A. I. Holleb and M. B. Randers-Pehrson, eds., *Classics in Oncology,* 137-138. New York: American Cancer Society, 1987.

Whitfield, M. L., et al. "Common Markers of Proliferation." *Nature Reviews Cancer* 6 (2006): 99-106.

Chapter 8: Get Prepared to Survive

April-Fritz, E. "Embracing My Life with Cancer." *Newsletter of the Whittingham Cancer Center at Norwalk Hospital* (Spring 2006): 6.

Gennaro, N., and M. Dailey. "Group of Survivors." *Newsletter of the Whittingham Cancer Center at Norwalk Hospital* (Spring 2006): 3.

Hermann, J. *Cancer Support Groups: A Guide for Facilitators.* New York: American Cancer Society, 2005.

Hewitt, M., and P. A. Ganz. *From Cancer Patient to Cancer Survivor: Lost in Transition.* Washington, DC: National Academies Press, 2006.

Silver, J. K. *After Cancer Treatment: Heal Faster, Better, Stronger.* Baltimore: Johns Hopkins University Press, 2006.

Taylor, P. "Survivors." *Newsletter of the Whittingham Cancer Center at Norwalk Hospital* (Spring 2006): 5.

Index

Page numbers in italics indicate illustrations